Practical ECG Holter

Jan Adamec · Richard Adamec
Hein J.J. Wellens

Practical ECG Holter

100 Cases

Foreword by François Mach

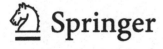 Springer

Jan Adamec, MD
av. du Casino 40
1820 Montreux
Switzerland
janadamec@bluewin.ch

Richard Adamec, MD
Che. Des Crets-de-Champel 33 1206
Geneva
Switzerland

Hein J.J. Wellens, MD
Professor of Cardiology
Maastricht University
Cardiovascular Research Institute Maastricht
21 Henric van Veldekeplein
6211 TG Maastricht
The Netherlands
hwellens@xs4all.nl

ISBN 978-1-4419-9954-2   e-ISBN 978-1-4419-9955-9
DOI 10.1007/978-1-4419-9955-9
Springer New York Dordrecht Heidelberg London

Library of Congress Control Number: 2011937622

Printed on acid-free paper

Springer is part of Springer Science+Business Media (www.springer.com)

Le Cœur

L'Amour le fait battre
Le sport le fait croître

Le vin rouge, il faut en boire
Pour plus longtemps pouvoir voir
Les splendeurs de la vie et
Le bonheur que procure les amis

Les désirs y sont enfouis

Le cœur a des maladies
Qui ne peuvent être guéries
Que par des médecins aguerris

Le cœur défie le temps
Au son de ses battements
                    K.A.

The Heart

Love makes it beat
The sport makes it grow

Red wine, we must drink
For longer to be able to see
The splendors of life and
The happiness that bring friends

The desires are hidden inside

The heart has diseases
Which can be cured
Only by experienced physicians

The heart defies the time
At the sound of its beating
                    K.A.

Grand-Puli

A Grand-Puli, pour qui la vie
N'a pas toujours été «easy»

De la médecine, tu as foulé le sentier
Pour en faire ton métier
A la perfection, tu l'as pratiqué

Tes fils et petits-enfants t'adorent
Ton cœur est d'or
Ta personnalité est attachante
Tes répliques sont foudroyantes

L'ironie, tu utilises avec génie
Ta générosité est innée
C'est pourquoi, ce soir, nous voulons te remercier

En t'offrant de modestes présents
Et en étant présents

Pour ce que tu nous as appris
Nous n'avons qu'un mot à dire:

Merci !
      K.A.

Grand-Puli

To Grand-Puli, for whom life
Has not always been easy

In medicine, you engaged yourself
To make it your profession
To the perfection, you have practiced it

Your sons and grandchildren adore you
Your heart is gold
Your personality is charming
Your replies are striking

The irony, you use brilliantly
Your generosity is inborn
Therefore, tonight, we want to thank you

By offering you a modest present
And by being present

For what you have taught us
We have only this to say:

Thank you!
      K.A.

For Maureen and Kilian
with the help of Aldebaran

Foreword

"Une vie toute tracée..."
"A predicable life line..."

Dr. Richard Adamec, in association with his son, Dr. Jan Adamec and Dr. Hein Wellens, proposes a new collection of quiz electrocardiographic (ECG) recordings. As may exist with certain kinds of pathologies, it seems there is a very important genetic predisposition to cardiology in this family, especially with regard to ECG interpretation.

It is quite evident that life expectancy increases and goes hand in hand with an increase in the number of cardiac beats during the complete life cycle. If the average heart rate is around 60 bpm, then a human's heart will experience more than three billion beats by the time he or she reaches the age of 80 years. As it is with most biological patterns, cardiac rhythm regularity may start to become less adequate with an increase in the number of beats. At a time when computers can interpret and outline an ECG diagnosis, you may ask yourself whether this new book proposed by Drs. Jan and Richard Adamec and Dr. Wellens is still relevant. Indeed, it is quite easy at any moment to receive and send ECG recordings from either our mobile phones or laptops. Nevertheless, we must note that a computer's interpretation of arrhythmias is still not performed very well, nor is it very accurate. For the time being, the human eye is still required and is much more reliable than any computer. In this field, we have not yet reached the same era as that in the game of chess, in which the best computer has beaten the human world chess champion.

The reading and the arrhythmia interpretation of a simple ECG is still very important for the treating physician. It is mandatory for the analysis to be very strict and for the physician to know all the clinical manifestations of the patient. For most physicians, the lectures and teaching about ECG recordings are quite timeworn, as they took place mostly during medical school. Nowadays, we know that the best way to relearn or brush up on our knowledge of something is through real-life experience. This book proposes exactly that, as it proceeds slide by slide through a rich variety of cases. Hence, it is an invitation to interpret the ECG recording and to rediscover its usefulness, not only for cardiologists but also for internal medicine specialists and general practitioners. The learning process is even more efficient when the problems presented are familiar. Sometimes it also is important to be challenged in order to learn even more; to achieve this aim, expert advice is always welcome.

I wish to thank Drs. Richard and Jan Adamec and Dr. Wellens for sharing their knowledge through these 100 ECG recordings. I am sure the readers will be very happy to revisit the basics, improve their knowledge, and through this, improve their skills.

Geneva, Switzerland

Professor François Mach
Chief-Physician
Cardiology Center
University Hospital of Geneva

Preface

Herewith is our new book of electrocardiography (ECG) tracings, all of which were collected on the shores of Lake Geneva, Switzerland. These 100 cases in no way comprise a new textbook or an ECG manual. By putting these 100 examples together, our intention is not to teach the basics of ECG. For this, many books are available, as well as plenty in your library, on the Internet, and on the shelves of your nearest university hospital library. The philosophy of this book is very different; it is based on the fact that most doctors use ECG in their medical practices to record tracings from their patients. Nevertheless, not many physicians have enough diversity of cases to stay sufficiently abreast of a wide variety of pathologies. Therefore, some lose proficiency in recognizing different ECG problems. The correct interpretation necessitates the knowledge we acquired first in medical school and relearned many times since – because we may have forgotten it many times. It also is very important to see real-life cases and to be exposed to many different problems. Thus, we came up with the idea of collecting 100 tracings from our clinical experience and sharing their interpretations with you, focusing on real-life cases. Of course, no book can present all possible ECG arrhythmias; therefore, we were obliged to make a selection among different problems. We limited ourselves to rhythm abnormalities because in this field, clinical ECG and Holter monitoring keep their unique value. In addition, the graphic limitation imposed by the page limit of this book obliged us to concentrate on problems that can be solved by a relatively short tracing.

Only a dependable diagnostic tool will allow a physician to make the correct diagnosis and consequently choose the correct treatment in case of an arrhythmia. However, that requires that the doctor feel comfortable when confronted with the interpretation of the ECG tracing. In presenting these tracings, we deliberately kept the cases as close to real life as possible. Thus, you will clearly feel that these tracings are indeed a collection from our practice and not hypothetical cases. Although the tracings might have been better presented with correct inscriptions and many diagrams, we refrained from including these because we believe presenting these arrhythmias in an atlas format might make the reader forget they can happen in ordinary life.

We have chosen to depict the tracings as we originally observed them, and we hope they will be of some help when in your practice, you have just recorded an ECG of a new patient. You will use your compass, or maybe only a piece of paper, to measure and compare the distances, and you will – we hope – react to these ECGs as you would on a daily basis. A big part of this collection is composed of tracings from Holter ECG recordings. This method, as well as the current use of event recorders, is very important and is the best available for arrhythmia diagnosis. Nevertheless, when interpreting ECG Holter recordings, please note that this method has some limitations. First, you must never forget that these tracings are obtained by two bipolar leads placed on the thorax. Because of this proximity, any movement of the chest or any difference in the projection of the heart during activities such as walking, running, or sleeping may modify their appearance. Therefore, very often the QRS complexes and the P waves are modified, even though there is a way to place the electrodes correctly. Very often in real life, you are obliged to place the leads where you can because of the thorax anatomy or just to be able to see QRS complexes or P waves of sufficient height. Because of the limitation of two or three leads, as well as their thoracic positioning, the frontal axis cannot be determined; therefore, not all the information from a standard 12-lead ECG can be gathered from a Holter recording. Moreover, we must keep in mind that correct ECG interpretation very often requires 12-lead clinical ECG, so interpretation of Holter monitoring should be applied with caution. Therefore, we cannot diagnose hypertrophies or ventricular dilatation or be certain about the type of bundle branch block, and so on.

Finally, Holter ECG may cause artifacts that may make the correct interpretation difficult or impossible. Before concluding that you are seeing a very peculiar arrhythmia, you must exclude any artifact. Likewise, before deciding that the phenomenon is an artifact, you should try to understand the mechanism, or even try to reproduce it.

Now, we would like to give you a few practical recommendations for a correct interpretation. First, it is important to determine the basic cardiac rhythm. On any tracing, you should first determine which of the following three situations is present:

1. The entire tracing is of sinus origin.
2. Some complexes are of sinus origin, but an arrhythmia also is present.
3. None of the complexes can be considered to be of sinus origin.

Therefore, it is of utmost importance to confirm or exclude sinus origin, to see how the sinus origin manifests itself at the atrial level and how it is conducted to the ventricular level. It therefore is also very important in the diagnosis of arrhythmias to determine the atrial activity as well as its origin: the ventricular complex may be the result of sinoatrial activity, ectopic atrial activity, or ectopic ventricular activity. Atrial activity or ventricular ectopic activity may appear prematurely, which is known as a premature beat. If the arrhythmic phenomenon occurs later, there must be a reason that prohibits the regular activity from manifesting itself. This situation usually requires the presence of either an escape complex or escape rhythm. This may be the result of a block at different levels, or a different arrhythmic phenomenon may be hidden or invisible and may remain blocked, producing this late phenomenon, as for instance with a blocked premature atrial beat.

An isolated abnormal phenomenon may be very difficult to interpret correctly, but once we see a repetition we may find logic in its appearance. This logic may become apparent by the frequency of appearances or its effect on the basic rhythm, as for example in the presence of a parasystole. When one or several wide QRS complexes occur, this abnormal phenomenon may be related to a rhythm frequency change, as for instance with frequency acceleration or deceleration during phase 3 or 4 blocks.

Sometimes to make a correct interpretation, you may only have to look at the distances of the previous complex and understand the phenomenon. In arrhythmias in which the atrial activity is not well seen or is seemingly absent, the presence of a regularity or irregularity may solve the problem. The irregularity may be completely irregular at the atrial level, as in atrial fibrillation, or regular at the atrial level but irregular at the ventricular level, as during an arrhythmia with fast atrial activity irregularly transmitted to the ventricles (e.g., in atrial flutter or atrial tachysystole). A regular irregularity in the presence of a slow heart rate should make us think of an irregular block at the sinoatrial level.

In case of an unusual bradycardia, one should consider a 2:1 atrioventricular block with hidden P waves in the previous T waves, an atrial blocked bigeminy, or a sinoatrial block.

After this brief introduction, we would like to let you discover the tracings, one by one, not necessarily in the order they are numbered, but in any order you like while turning the pages of our book.

For more explanation, we recommend for reference the *ECG Holter Guide to Electrocardiographic Interpretation* by Jan and Richard Adamec, published by Springer, and *The ECG in Emergency Decision Making*, second edition, by Hein Wellens and Mary Conover, published by Elsevier. These books will help you understand the different tracings; especially with regard to the difficult cases, we recommend you read them beforehand.

We wish you a pleasant adventure.

Clarens-Montreux, Switzerland   Jan Adamec
Geneva, Switzerland   Richard Adamec
Maastricht, The Netherlands   Hein J.J. Wellens

Contents

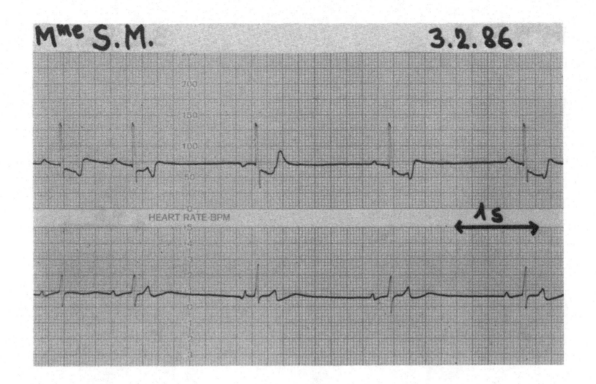

ECG no. 101: Mrs. S.M., 84 years

Repetitive episodes of syncope
ECG Holter recording

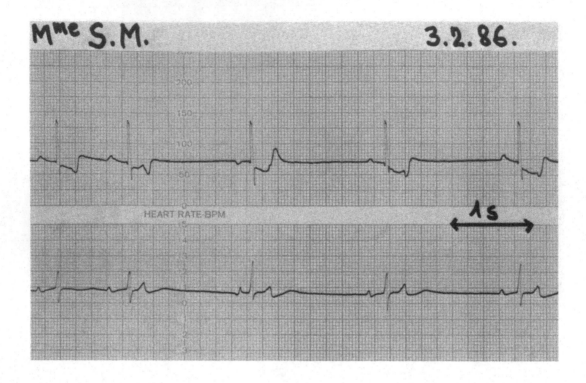

ECG no. 101: Mrs. S.M., 84 years

ECG Holter recording

The first two complexes are of sinus origin. In the repolarization phase of the second QRS, there is an atrial premature beat that is not conducted to the ventricle. This provokes a post-extrasystolic pause terminated by an escape of atrial origin (negative P wave) that is conducted to the ventricle. A new ectopic P′ wave hidden in the repolarization phase of the QRS is also blocked and causes a new post-extrasystolic pause terminated by a sinus beat. A similar sequence of events is repeated thereafter.

Conclusion

Blocked atrial bigeminy.

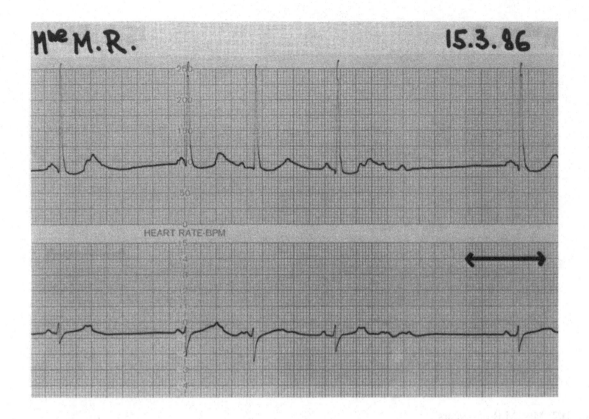

ECG no. 102: Mrs. M.R., 56 years

Palpitations, malaise
ECG Holter recording

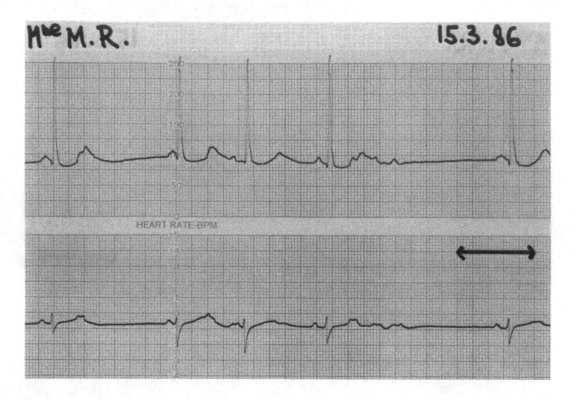

HEART RATE BPM

ECG no. 102: Mrs. M.R., 56 years

ECG Holter recording

   The first complex is a conducted sinus beat. In the T wave of the first QRS, there is a blocked atrial premature beat. The second QRS is preceded by a sinus P wave that is situated too close to the ventricular complex to be conducted. In and shortly after the T wave of the second QRS, two P waves are present, the second of which is conducted to the ventricle. In and after the repolarization phase of the fourth QRS, we find three ectopic P′ waves, which are all blocked to the ventricle. The pause is terminated by a conducted sinus beat.

Conclusion

   Repetitive atrial ectopic activity, often not conducted to the ventricle, with a short episode of atrial tachycardia.

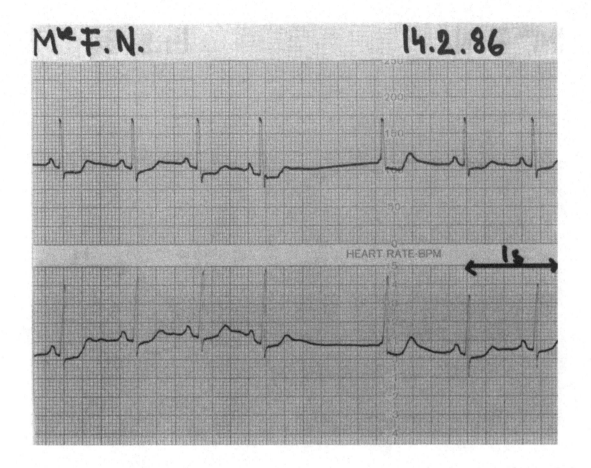

ECG no. 103: Mrs. F.N., 69 years

Palpitations, malaise
ECG Holter recording

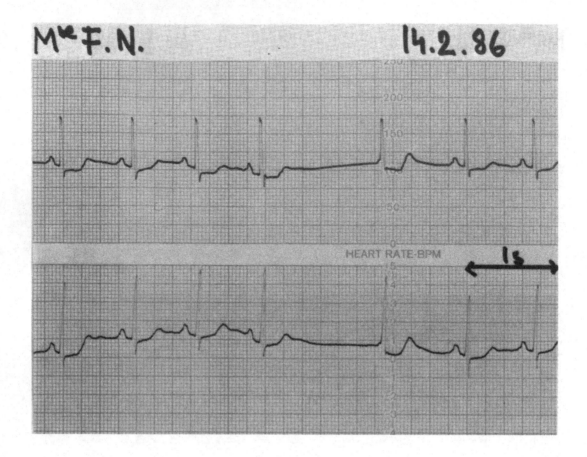

ECG no. 103: Mrs. F.N., 69 years

ECG Holter recording

   Normal sinus rhythm. Four almost identical P–P and R–R intervals are followed by a pause, which is exactly double the P–P interval. The pause terminates with a junctional escape with the sinus P wave halfway in the R wave. The last two complexes are conducted sinus beats.

Conclusion

   Typical second-degree sinoatrial block of the Mobitz-2 type.

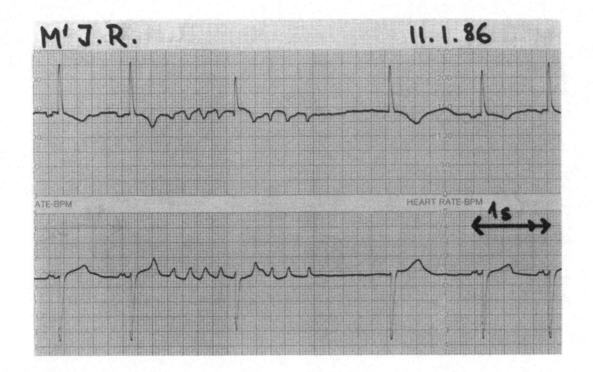

ECG no. 104: Mr. J.R., 74 years

History of myocardial infarction
History of atrial fibrillation and flutter, digoxin, amiodarone
ECG Holter recording

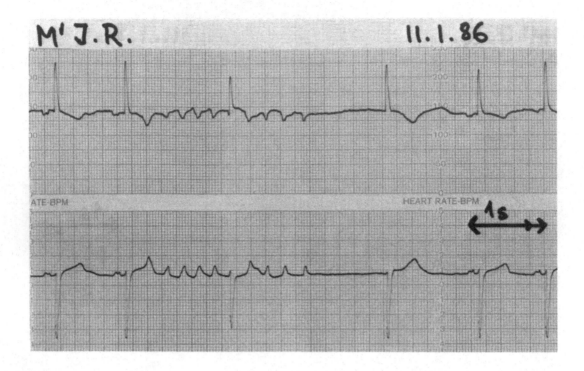

ECG no. 104: Mr. J.R., 74 years

ECG Holter recording

The first two QRS are preceded by a P wave of unidentifiable origin (negative in the upper lead!). After the second QRS, fast irregular atrial activity is present – on average, 280 bpm – suggesting atrial tachycardia. This activity lasts for 2.2 s, with only one ventricular complex. This fast atrial activity stops, and the pause is terminated by a junctional escape.

Conclusion

Atrial tachycardia lasting only 2.2 s.

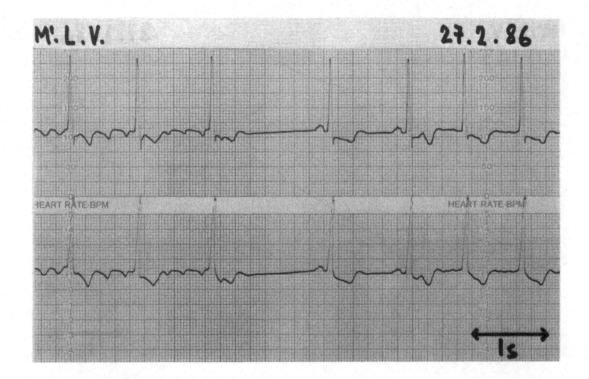

ECG no. 105: Mr. L.V., 73 years

History of atrial fibrillation and flutter
ECG Holter recording

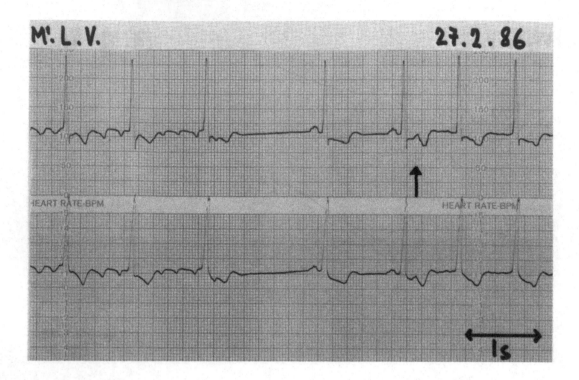

ECG no. 105: Mr. L.V., 73 years

ECG Holter recording

The first three ventricular complexes are preceded by fast atrial activity (~250 bpm), suggesting atrial flutter with 4:1 and 5:1 ventricular conduction. The atrial activity accelerates and stops during the repolarization phase of the third QRS. Thereafter, two conducted sinus P waves are present; in the T wave of the second one, we can identify an atrial extrasystole (↑), which causes atrial fibrillation. The last two ventricular complexes are preceded by atrial fibrillation.

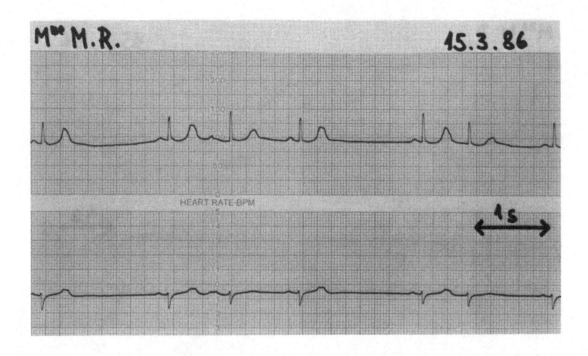

ECG no. 106: Mrs. M.R., 56 years

Malaise
ECG Holter recording

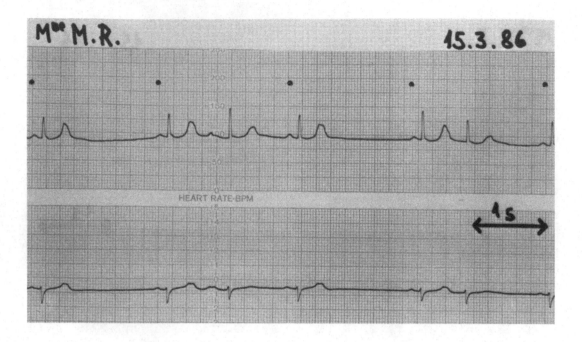

ECG no. 106: Mrs. M.R., 56 years

ECG Holter recording

Cardiac activity is irregular and interrupted by pauses. Some P waves have sinus morphology (•); their appearance is regular but slow (~34 bpm). The ventricular complexes are all narrow and have the same morphology. However, the T waves are not all the same. The T waves in the third and sixth ventricular complexes seem normal (particularly in the lower lead), but in the other T waves (from the first, second, fourth, and fifth complexes) an ectopic P′ wave is present. The ectopic P′ wave after the first complex is blocked and provokes a post-extrasystolic pause. After the second complex, we find two ectopic P′ waves, the first one blocked and the second one conducted to the ventricle. The ectopic P′ wave following the fourth complex is again blocked and followed by a post-extrasystolic pause. The ectopic P′ wave following the fifth ventricular complex conducts to the ventricles.

Conclusion

Often blocked atrial extrasystoles resulting in a ventricular bradycardia.

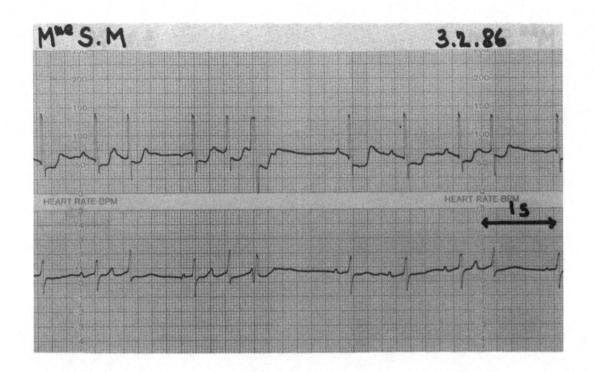

ECG no. 107: Mrs. S.M., 84 years

Multiple episodes of syncope
ECG Holter recording

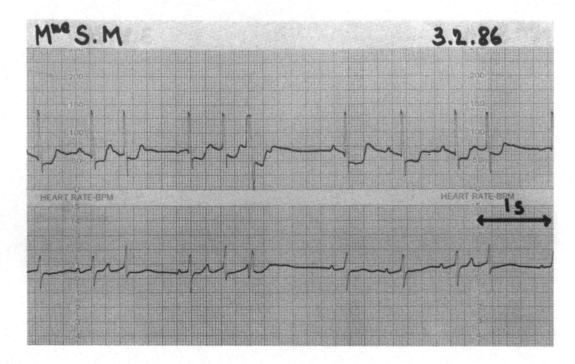

ECG no. 107: Mrs. S.M., 84 years

ECG Holter recording

The first two complexes are of sinus origin. Then, we see a premature atrial beat in the T wave of the previous QRS. The atrial premature beat is conducted to the ventricle with a slightly different QRS (best seen in the lower recording), most likely because of aberrant intraventricular conduction. Following the pause, there are three ventricular complexes, probably conducted from an ectopic atrial rhythm. The last QRS is widest (0.12 s), probably because of more aberrant conduction. In the repolarization phase of this QRS, there is a new ectopic P′ wave and then three conducted sinus beats, and a new atrial extrasystole. The last complex is another atrial escape.

Conclusion

Atrial extrasystoles. The wide QRS likely is of atrial origin with aberrant intraventricular conduction.

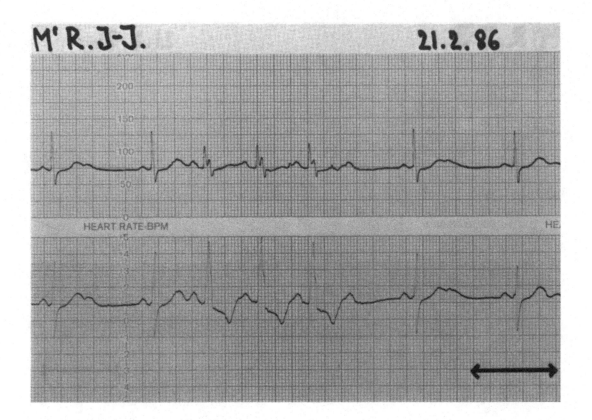

ECG no. 108: Mr. R.J.-J., 70 years

Fatigue
Breathlessness
ECG Holter recording

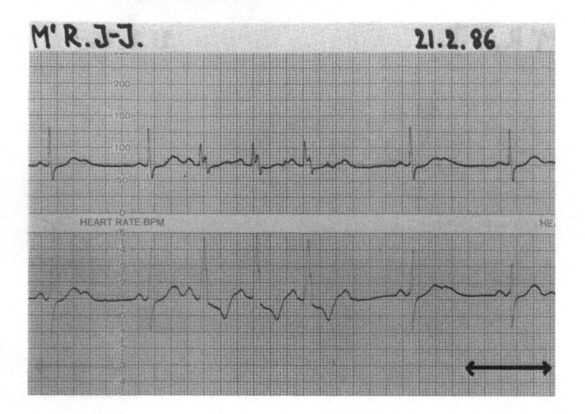

ECG no. 108: Mr. R.J.-J., 70 years

ECG Holter recording

The first QRS is a conducted sinus beat. The P wave following the T wave does not conduct. The third P wave conducts with a narrow QRS complex. The following three P waves, which are slightly different from the sinus P wave, are conducted to the ventricle, but with a wider QRS complex. This QRS widening most likely is caused by rate-related interventricular aberrant conduction. The P wave after the last widened QRS is again blocked and then followed by a conducted sinus beat with a narrow QRS complex. The P wave after that is also blocked. The last P wave conducts again with a narrow QRS complex.

Conclusion

Frequent conducted and nonconducted ectopic atrial beats with rate-related QRS widening due to aberrant interventricular conduction.

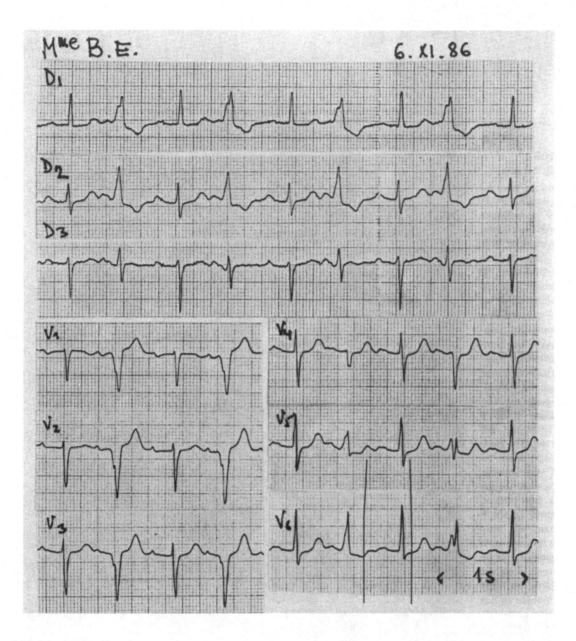

ECG no. 109: Mrs. B.E., 68 years

Hypertension, ischemic heart disease
Heart insufficiency; treatment: digoxin, 1 pill 5 days/week, and diuretics

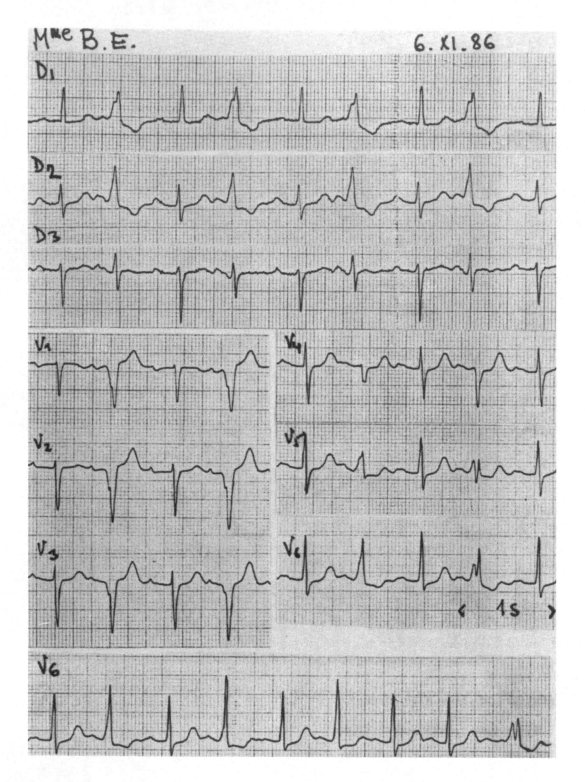

ECG no. 109: Mrs. B.E., 68 years

The basic rhythm is sinus rhythm. The narrow QRS complexes are conducted sinus beats (the first, third, fifth, seventh, and ninth complexes). The PR interval measures 0.24 s, the frontal QRS axis is around −30°, and the QRS lasts for 80 ms. The conducted sinus beats are followed by a wide ventricular complex (120 ms) with the appearance of a left bundle branch block (QS in V_1 and wide R in V_6). These wide QRS complexes are preceded by a P wave but with a shorter PR interval (~0.20 s), suggesting ventricular bigeminy, originating – because of their left bundle branch block-like configuration – in the right ventricle. The ventricular premature beats (VPBs) occur late after the P wave with some fusion with the conducted sinus beat, which is more or less present. This is seen clearly in leads V_4 through V_6 at the bottom of the page, where the fusion is most marked in the first extrasystole (second QRS complex).

Conclusion

Sinus rhythm with ventricular bigeminy, arising in the right ventricle.

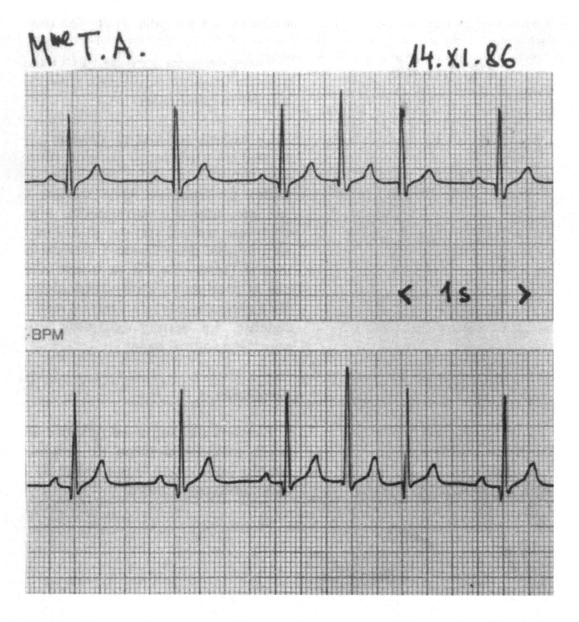

ECG no. 110: Ms. T.A., 24 years

Palpitations, no treatment
ECG Holter recording

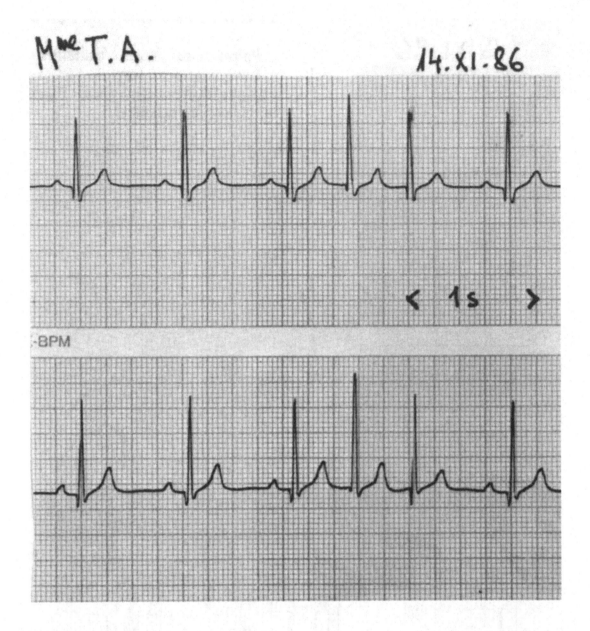

ECG no. 110: Ms. T.A., 24 years

ECG Holter recording

The conducted sinus beats are interrupted by a premature supraventricular beat with a narrow QRS. There is PR prolongation of the conducted sinus P wave following this premature beat because of concealed AV conduction produced by the preceding extrasystole.

Conclusion

Interpolated supraventricular extrasystole with concealed AV conduction.

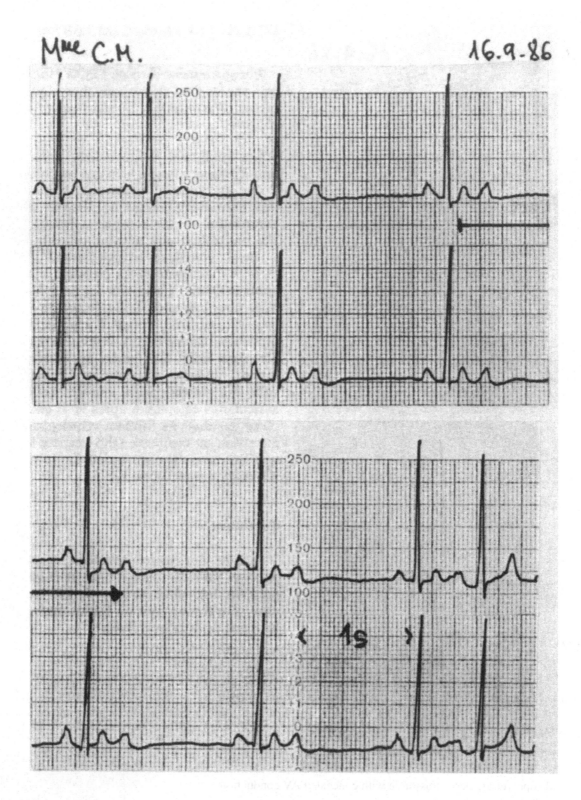

ECG no. 111: Mrs. C.M., 68 years

Palpitations, dyspnea
Treatment: digoxin, 1 pill 5 days/week, and quinidine arabogalactane sulfate, 2 pills per day
ECG Holter recording

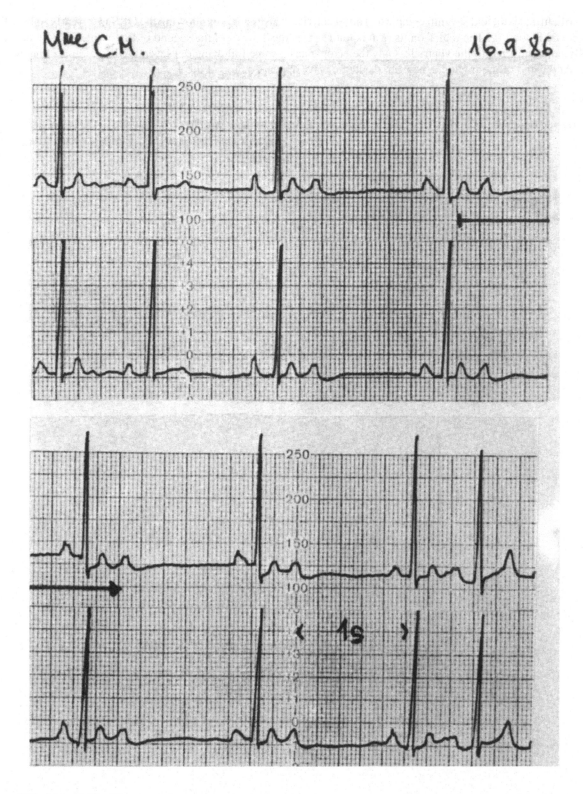

ECG no. 111: Mrs. C.M., 68 years

ECG Holter recording

Continuous recording

   The ventricular complexes do appear to be of sinus origin even though the P waves preceding them have a peculiar morphology. In the repolarization phase of these complexes (except the second one), we find isolated (first complex) or repetitive

23

(third, fourth, fifth, sixth, and seventh complexes) atrial activity. The first wave following the QRS is too early to be a T wave, and the second is too big. The real T on its own is flatter, as is the T wave of the second QRS complex. These atrial waves are usually not conducted to the ventricle. Only the ectopic atrial wave following the seventh QRS complex conducts to the ventricle. At the end of the tracing, a new atrial ectopic wave appears on top of the T wave.

Conclusion

Repetitive ectopic atrial activity, which is usually not conducted to the ventricle.

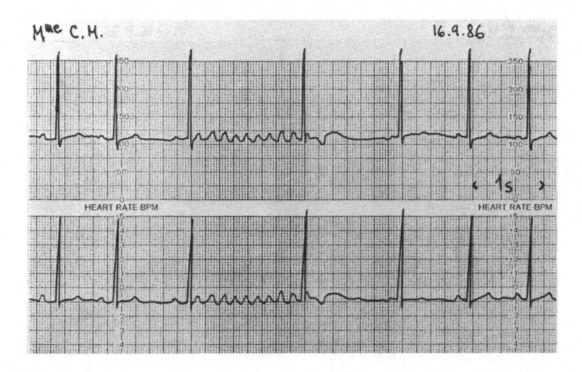

HEART RATE BPM

HEART RATE BPM

ECG no. 112: Mrs. C.M., 68 years

Palpitations, dyspnea
Treatment: digoxin, 1 pill 5 days/week, and quinidine arabogalactane sulfate, 2 pills per day
ECG Holter recording

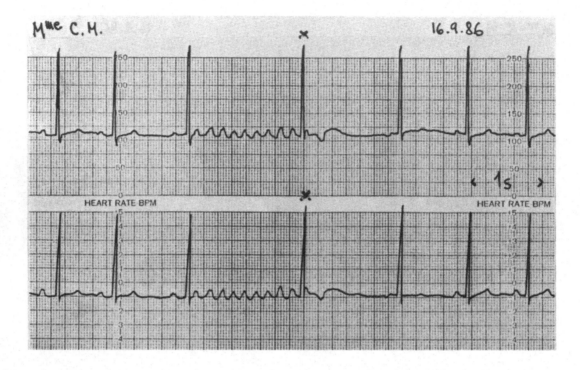

ECG no. 112: Mrs. C.M., 68 years

ECG Holter recording

Sinus rhythm (the first three complexes) slows down and is interrupted by fast atrial activity (~350 bpm). This atrial rhythm is not completely regular, as evidenced by waves of variable morphologies. This rapid atrial rhythm has a ventricular complex (X) at the end. In its repolarization phase (ST segment), the atrial activity stops. The next complex, because of its negative P wave, is not of sinus origin; it is a low atrial or junctional escape beat. The last two complexes of the tracing are of sinus origin.

Conclusion

Onset of fast ectopic atrial activity lasting no longer than 1.5 s. Its frequency – more than 350 bpm – suggests an episode of atrial fibrillation. The rhythm change, before and after onset with the presence of an escape rhythm, makes an artifact unlikely.

26

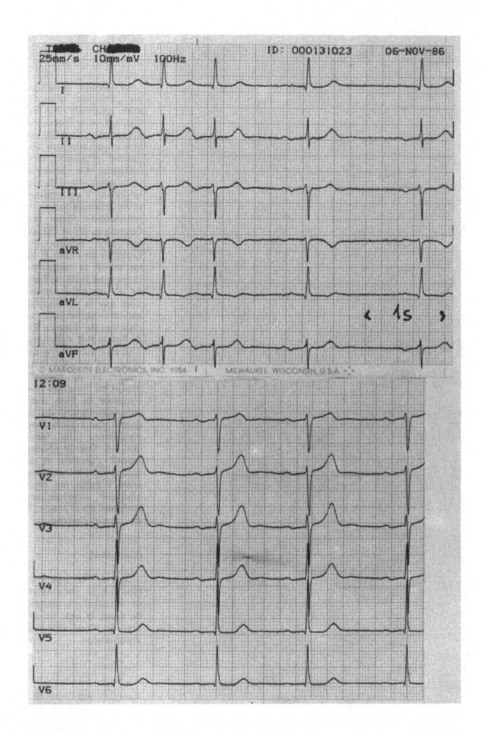

ECG no. 113: Mr. I.C.H., 70 years

Multiple episodes of presyncope
No treatment

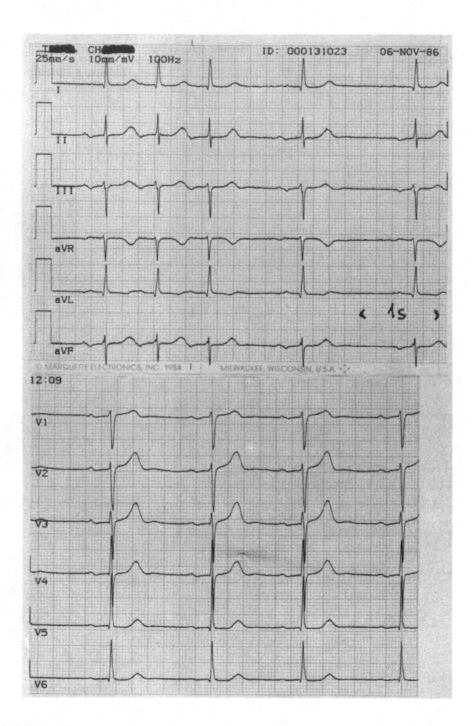

ECG no. 113: Mr. I.C.H., 70 years

The first three complexes are conducted sinus beats with a prolonged PQ interval of 0.28 s. The P wave in leads II and III is biphasic with terminal negativity. This negativity at the end of the T wave is also visible in leads II and III preceding the second and third QRS. Following the third QRS, there is a pause that is terminated with a conducted sinus P wave. The interval between this P wave and the P wave before QRS three is exactly twice the P–P interval preceding QRS 2 and 3, indicating the presence of 2:1 sinoatrial block. This persists in the following beats.

Conclusion

2:1 Sinoatrial block and prolonged AV nodal conduction.

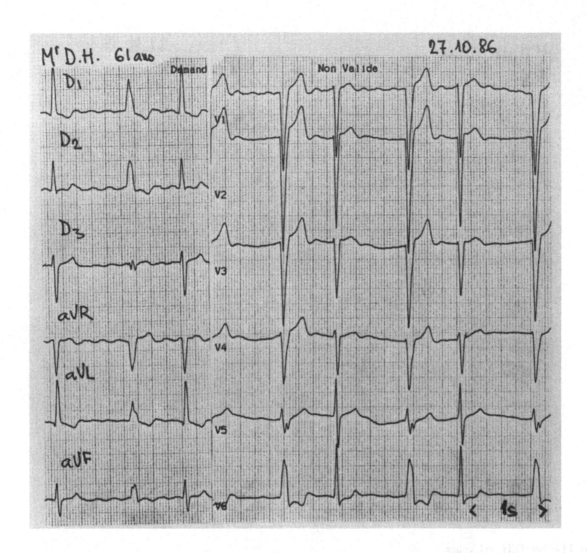

ECG no. 114: Mr. D.H., 61 years

Arterial hypertension, chronic coronary disease; digoxin, 1 pill per day, and diuretics

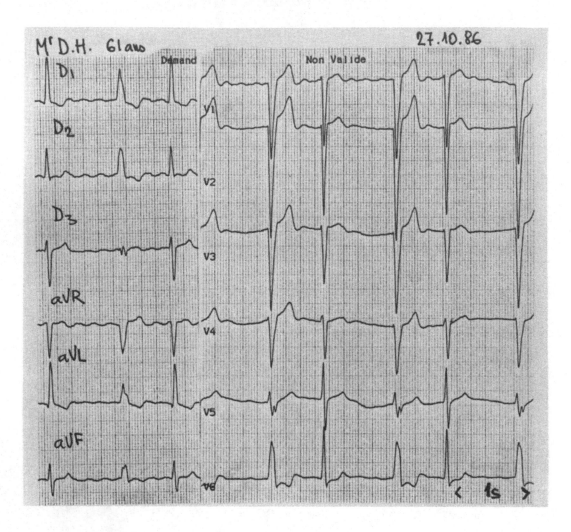

ECG no. 114: Mr. D.H., 61 years

At the atrial level, a regular rhythm is present with a rate of around 260 bpm, suggesting atrial flutter. The ventricular complexes have two morphologies: one is narrow (100 ms), and the other is wide (120 ms). The interval between the two ventricular complexes (R–R) is either long (1,000 ms) or short (730 ms). The narrow complex always appears after the short interval, and the wide complex always appears after the long interval. The alternating R–R interval may be explained by a two-level block in the AV conduction system: a 3:2 Wenckebach block in the upper level and a 2:1 block in the lower level. For the occurrence of the wide QRS after the long R–R interval, two possibilities must be considered: either phase 4 block in the left bundle branch or an escape arising in the right ventricle. The QRS characteristics during the wide QRS speak in favor of phase 4 block.

Conclusion

Atrial flutter with variable AV conduction because of a two-level block in the AV conduction system, resulting in an alternating R–R interval length. The left bundle branch block aberration after the long R–R interval may be explained by phase 4 block in the left bundle branch.

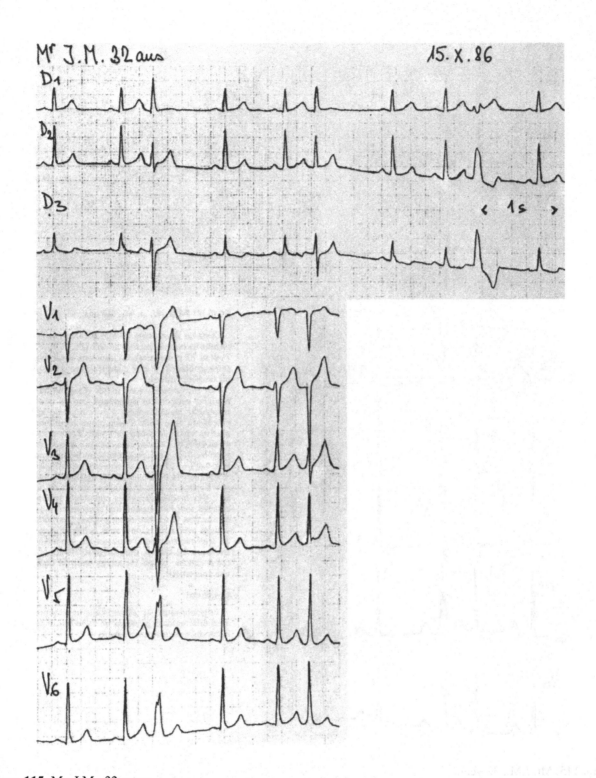

Mr J.M. 32 ans   15.X.86

ECG no. 115: Mr. J.M., 32 years

Palpitations
No known heart disease
No treatment

31

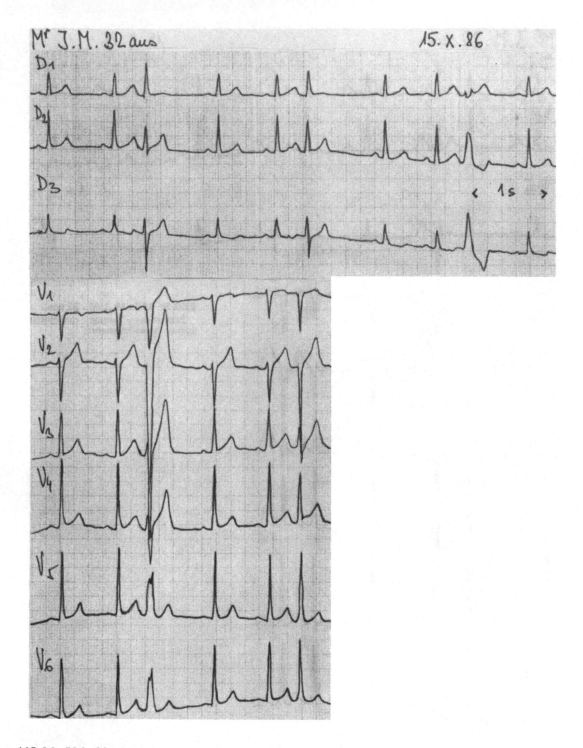

ECG no. 115: Mr. J.M., 32 years

In the *upper panel*, leads I, II, and III show conducted sinus beats (the first, second, fourth, fifth, seventh, eighth, and tenth complexes). This rhythm is interrupted by premature beats (third, sixth, and ninth complexes), suggesting trigeminy. Although they are wide, all these premature beats are of atrial origin, as evidenced by the T wave preceding the complexes where the

32

ectopic P' waves can be recognized. The QRS complex of the premature beat changes; it is narrow for the first two, but the axis changes (−15° for the first premature beat, +30° for the second). The third premature QRS complex widens, and its morphology suggests left bundle branch block with an axis of +90°. These modifications of the ventricular complexes are an expression of aberrant intraventricular conduction. In the precordial leads, we find the same trigeminy.

Conclusion

Trigeminy due to atrial premature beats. There are different degrees of left-sided aberrant conductions.

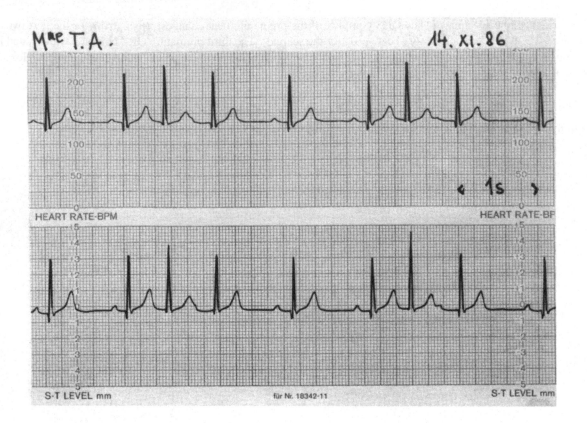

ECG no. 116: Mrs. T.A.

Palpitations
Holter ECG recording

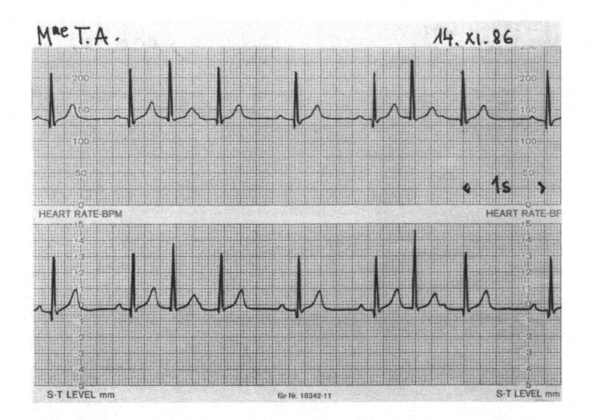

ECG no. 116: Mrs. T.A.

Holter ECG recording

The basic rhythm is a sinus rhythm, quite slow at 60 bpm. The sinus P wave precedes the first, second, fifth, sixth, and ninth QRS complexes. Following the second and sixth QRS complexes, interpolated premature beats are present. They have a narrow QRS and are not preceded by a P wave, suggesting an AV junctional origin. They are followed by a prolonged PR interval of the next conducted sinus beat. The PR prolongation is caused by retrograde AV nodal invasion by the junctional premature beat.

Conclusion

Supraventricular interpolated extrasystoles with retrograde "concealed" conduction in the AV node.

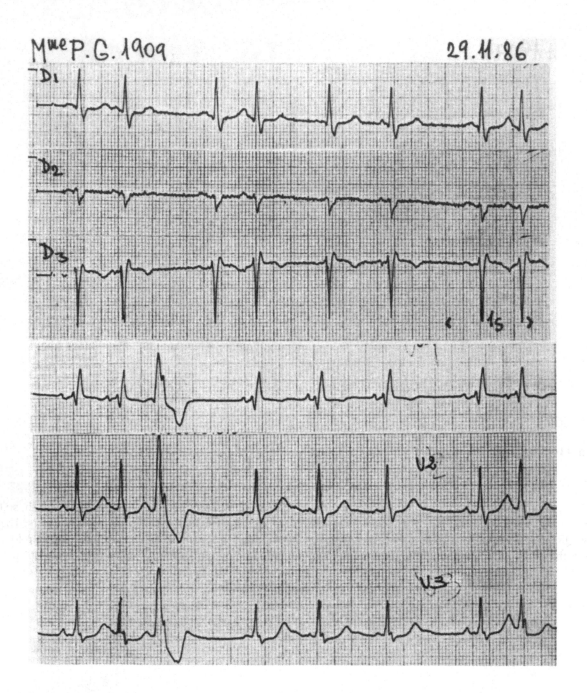

ECG no. 117: Mrs. P.G., 78 years

Cardiac insufficiency
Chronic digoxin treatment

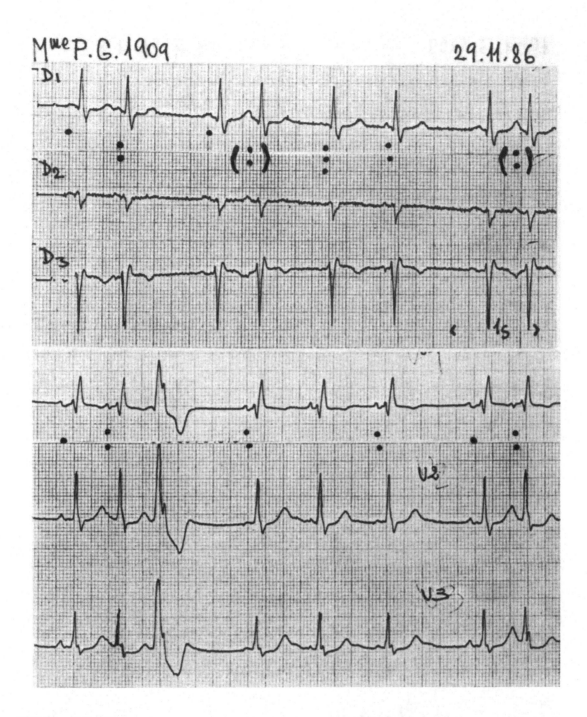

ECG no. 117: Mrs. P.G., 78 years

Leads I, II, and III show irregular cardiac activity. All the ventricular complexes are identical and wide (120 ms), showing right bundle branch block with left anterior hemiblock. The atrial activity presents P waves of different morphologies. Both sinus rhythm and ectopic atrial activity are present. The precordial leads show a VPB (third QRS complex). The second, third, fifth, and seventh P′ waves (:) have the same morphology, and the intervals separating them are identical (1.52 s), suggesting the possibility of an atrial parasystole.

Conclusion

We are in the presence of atrial hyperexcitability due to a low potassium level and digitalis intoxication, possibly presenting an atrial parasystole.

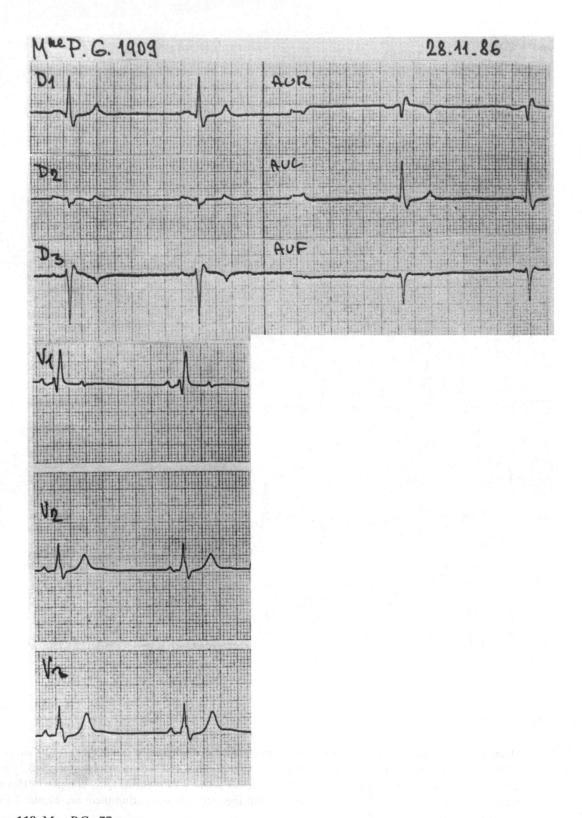

ECG no. 118: Mrs. P.G., 77 years

Cardiac insufficiency
Chronic digoxin treatment
Diuretics

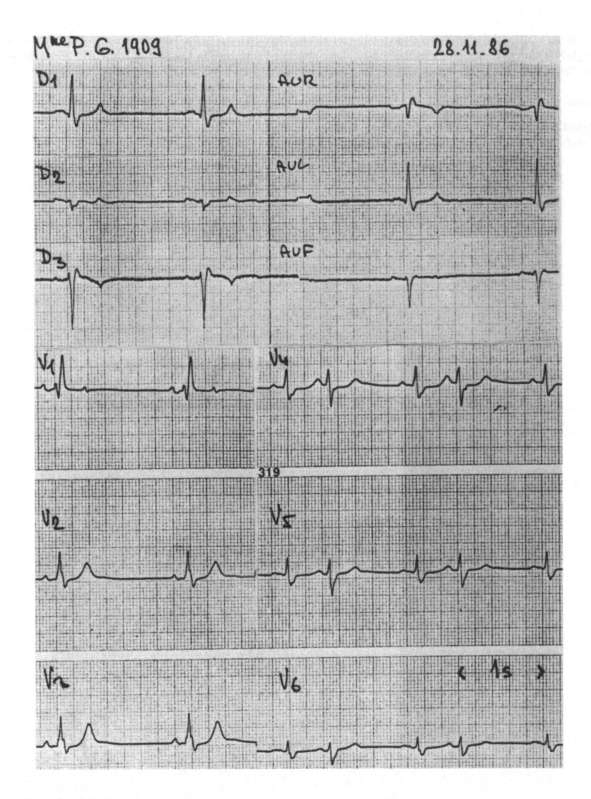

ECG no. 118: Mrs. P.G., 77 years

At first glance, it looks like a sinus bradycardia at 40 bpm, but the bradycardia due to blocked atrial premature beats in bigeminy. The ectopic P′ wave hidden in the T wave of the previous conducted sinus beat is well seen in leads III and V₁. The QRS complex shows right bundle branch block with left anterior hemiblock. In the left precordial leads shown on the next page, the atrial extrasystoles are no longer blocked and conduct to the ventricles with a QRS complex showing a slightly different morphology as the ventricular complex of sinus origin because of some additional delay in the posterior fascicle.

Conclusion

- Transiently blocked atrial bigeminy mimicking sinus bradycardia.
- Complete right bundle branch block with left anterior hemiblock.

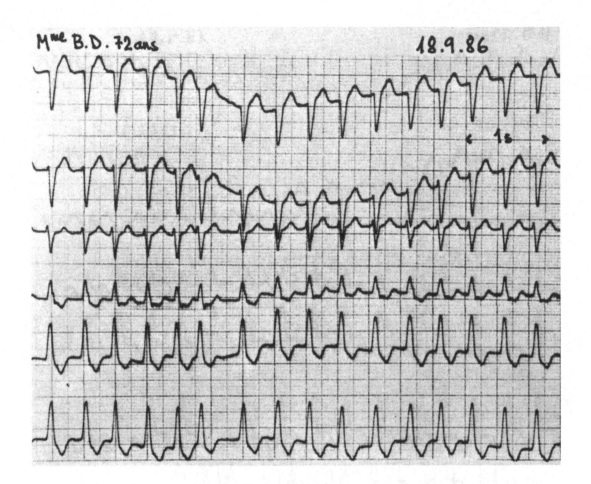

ECG no. 119: Mrs. B.D., 72 years

Coronary artery disease
Shortness of breath
Heart failure
Digoxin
Diuretics

41

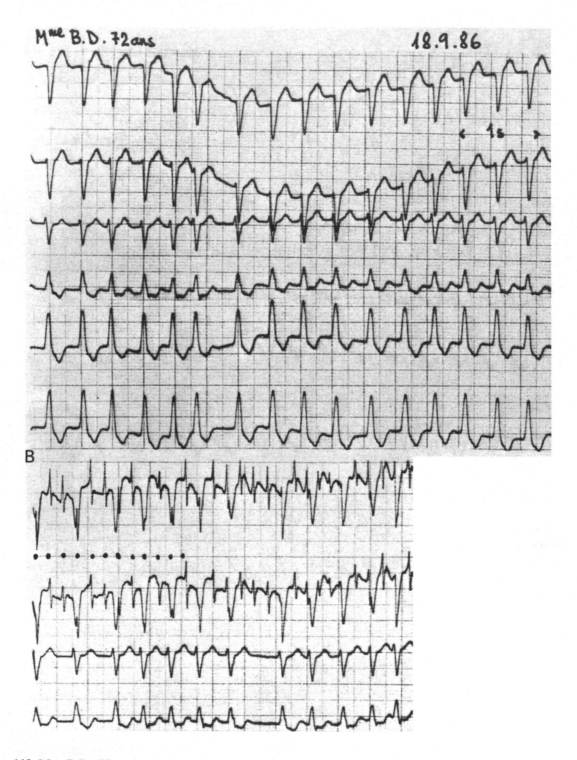

ECG no. 119: Mrs. B.D., 72 years

Fast and irregular ventricular rhythm; the ventricular complex presents the morphology of left bundle branch block. The atrial activity is not seen on the upper part of the tracing, and a relative irregularity should make us think of a probable atrial fibrillation. In the bottom part of the tracing (B), the first two leads represent an esophageal recording via a unipolar lead. We clearly see a fast atrial activity (340 bpm) that is regular (•); therefore, we are in the presence of atrial flutter with variable conduction to the ventricles.

NB: This example shows the usefulness of an esophageal recording, which is not as difficult to perform as usually imagined; it can be performed easily with a provisional pacing lead.

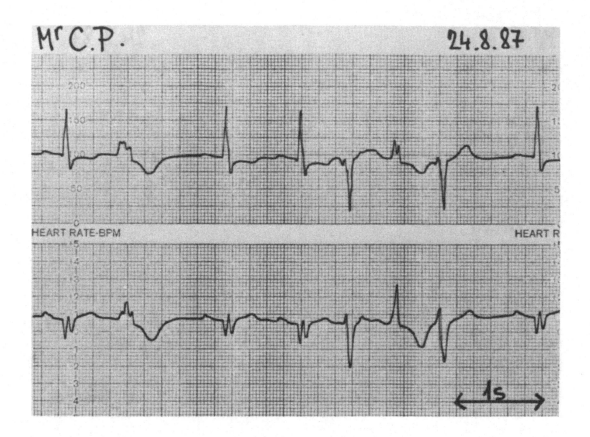

ECG no. 120: Mr. C.P., 75 years

Coronary artery disease
Heart failure
Paroxysmal nightly dyspnea
Furosemide, enalapril, oral nitrate
Holter ECG recording

43

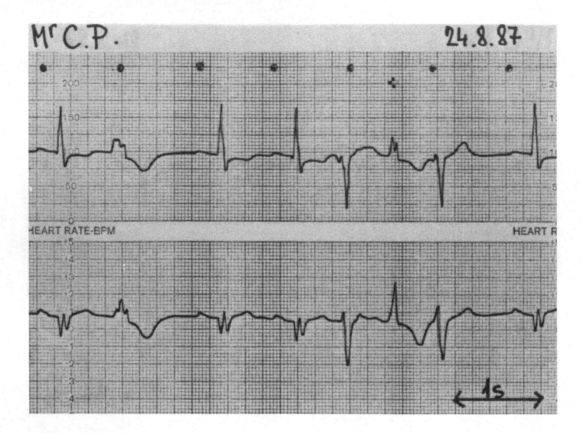

ECG no. 120: Mr. C.P., 75 years

Holter ECG recording

Sinus rhythm at the atrial level, with P waves present at regular intervals (•) and a prolonged PR interval. The first conducted sinus complex is followed by a wide QRS premature beat. After a fully compensatory pause, there are two conducted sinus beats and then three beats with a wide QRS complex showing QRS alternation. After a pause, a conducted sinus beat terminates the recording.

Conclusion

Ventricular extrasystoles with different QRS morphologies.

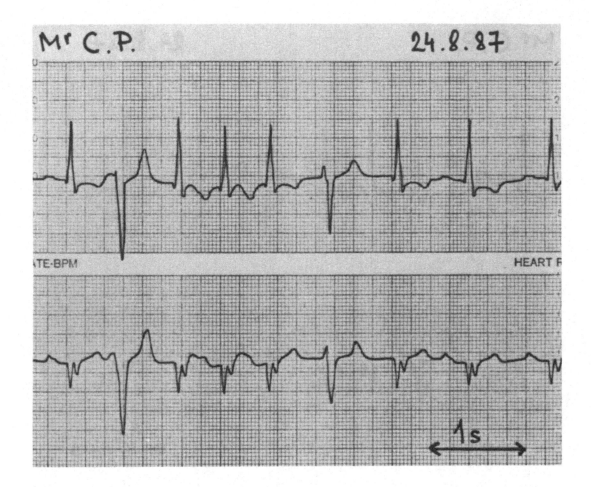

ECG no. 121: Mr. C.P., 75 years

Coronary disease
Heart failure
Paroxysmal nightly dyspnea; furosemide, enalapril, oral nitrate
Holter ECG recording

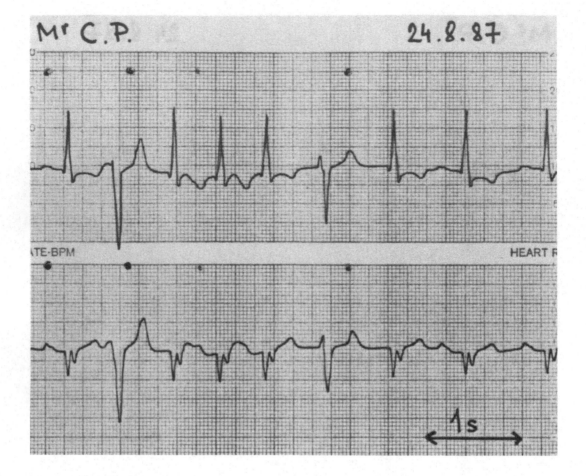

ECG no. 121: Mr. C.P., 75 years

Holter ECG recording

The first complex is a conducted sinus beat; the second is a wide QRS premature beat followed by a new sinus beat with the P wave hidden in the extrasystolic T wave (•). The next complex is also of sinus origin. The complex thereafter is a conducted atrial extrasystole. The following wide QRS complex is a premature ventricular beat. We then have three conducted sinus beats, the P wave of the first complex being hidden in the extrasystolic T wave. The lengthening in AV conduction (PR interval) in beats 3 and 7 is the result of retrograde concealed conduction by the VPB.

Conclusion

The irregularity of the rhythm is the result of two VPBs and one supraventricular premature beat.

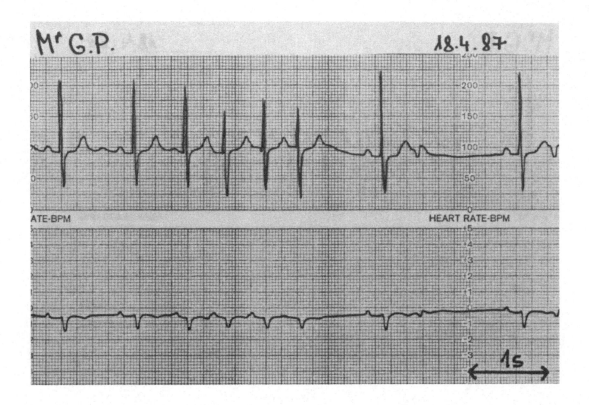

ECG no. 122: Mr. G.P., 76 years

Vertigo
Malaise
Holter ECG recording

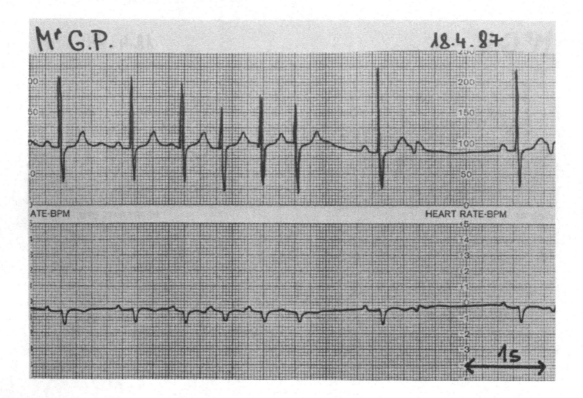

ECG no. 122: Mr. G.P., 76 years

Holter ECG recording

The first two complexes are conducted sinus beats. They are followed by an atrial tachycardia of four complexes with a heart rate of 120 bpm. Thereafter, a conducted sinus beat is followed by a blocked atrial extrasystole, a conducted sinus P wave, and finally an atrial extrasystole.

Conclusion

Atrial tachycardia and early atrial premature beats not conducted to the ventricle.

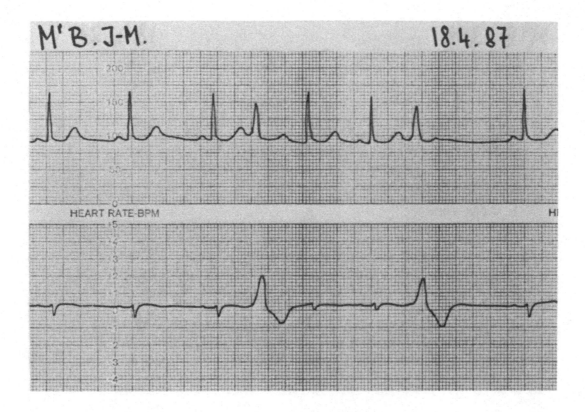

ECG no. 123: Mr. B.J.-M., 55 years

Retrosternal chest pain
Palpitations
Holter ECG recording

49

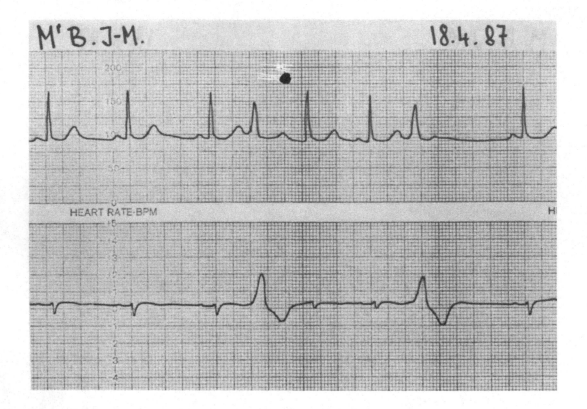

ECG no. 123: Mr. B.J.-M., 55 years

Holter ECG recording

The first three complexes are of sinus origin. Then there is a VPB and two narrow QRS complexes preceded by a sinus P wave. Then we have a new VPB and, following a pause, a conducted sinus P wave. The first VPB is interpolated between two conducted sinus complexes; the P wave of the post-extrasystolic complex is hidden in the T wave (•), and the PR interval is prolonged because of concealed retrograde AV nodal penetration by the VPB. The second VPB occurs a little later, resulting in AV block of the sinus P wave.

Conclusion

An example of PR prolongation and AV block, depending on the timing of the VPB.

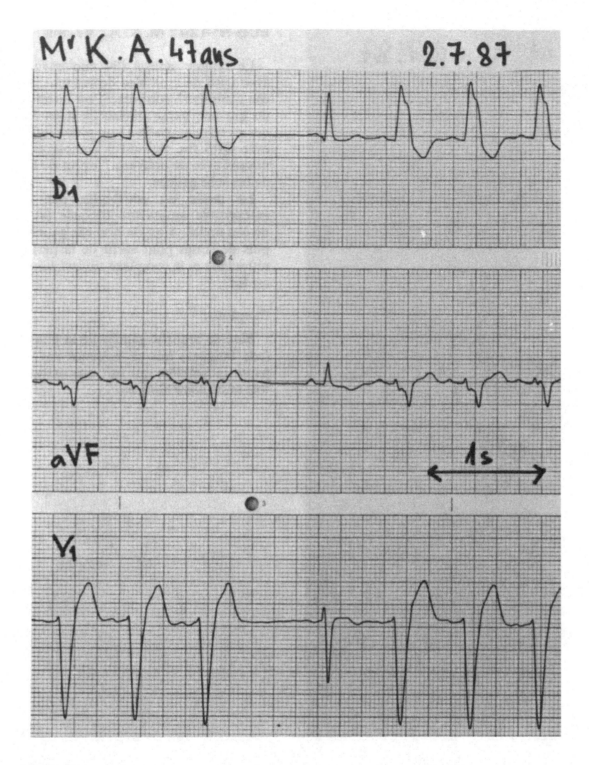

ECG no. 124: Mr. K.A., 47 years

Aortic valve disease
Exercise-induced shortness of breath

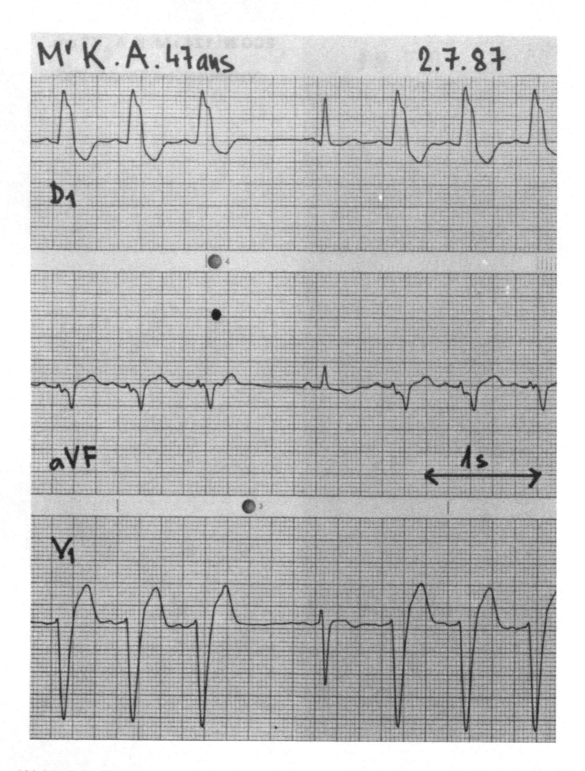

ECG no. 124: Mr. K.A., 47 years

The sinus tachycardia (95 bpm) has a QRS morphology of complete left bundle branch block (three complexes) and is interrupted by a pause that is terminated by a sinus beat with a narrow QRS. Thereafter, three QRS complexes with left bundle branch block are present. The pause is caused by a blocked atrial premature beat (•) best seen in lead aVF. This is an example of acceleration-dependent left bundle branch block, with bundle branch block occurring at a rate of 95 bpm. It should not be called phase 3 block, which occurs at much faster rates and is a precursor of complete bundle branch block.

Conclusion

Acceleration-dependent left bundle branch block, diagnosed with the help of a pause following a blocked atrial extrasystole.

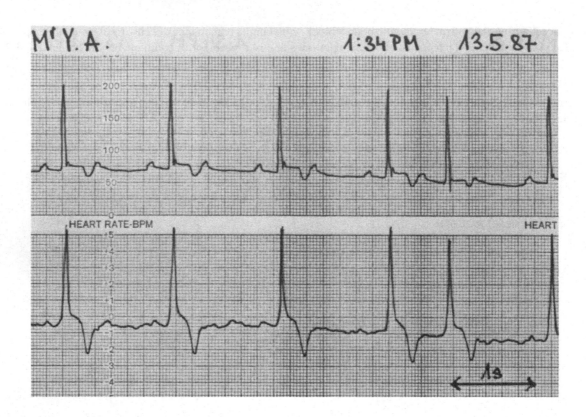

ECG no. 125: Mr. Y.A., 69 years

Coronary artery disease
Palpitations
Malaise
Holter ECG recording

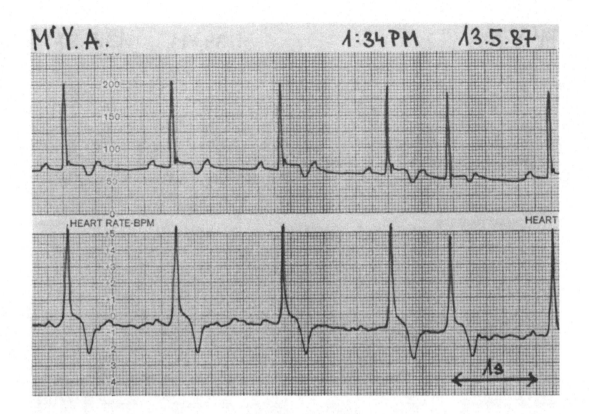

ECG no. 125: Mr. Y.A., 69 years

Holter ECG recording

The first four QRS complexes are preceded by two sinus P waves, indicating 2:1 AV block. At the end of the recording, a 3:2 Wenckebach-type second-degree AV block is present.

Conclusion

Second-degree AV block type 2:1 and type Wenckebach.

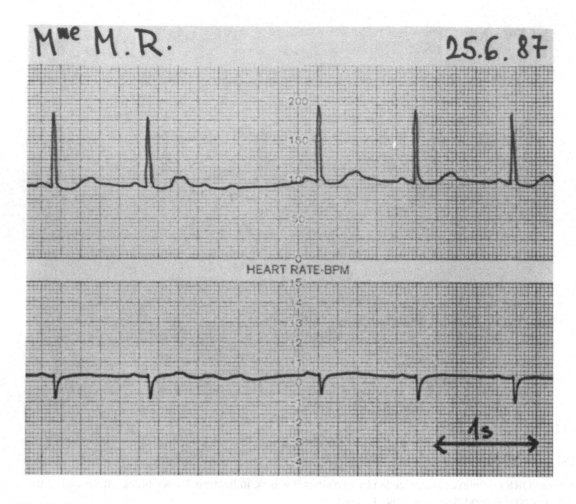

ECG no. 126: Mrs. M.R., 57 years

Palpitations
Holter ECG recording

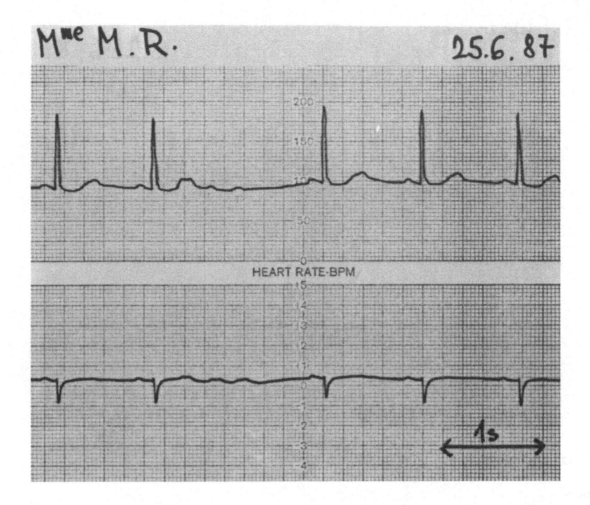

ECG no. 126: Mrs. M.R., 57 years

Holter ECG recording

Normal sinus rhythm is interrupted by three beats of ectopic atrial activity with a heart rate of around 240 bpm, suggesting atrial tachycardia. All three ectopic P′ waves are blocked; following a pause, we again see sinus P waves, followed by narrow QRS complexes identical to the first two. However, the PR interval of the first post-pause beat is too short to be a conducted sinus beat. Therefore, that QRS represents an AV junctional escape.

Conclusion

Blocked atrial tachycardia (three P′ waves) followed by a junctional escape.

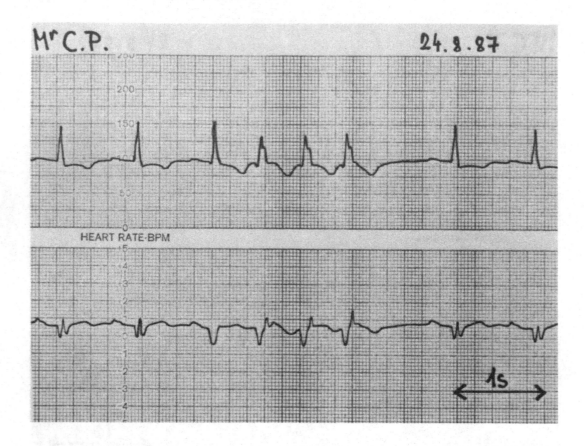

ECG no. 127: Mr. C.P., 75 years

Palpitations
Coronary artery disease
Heart failure
Holter ECG recording

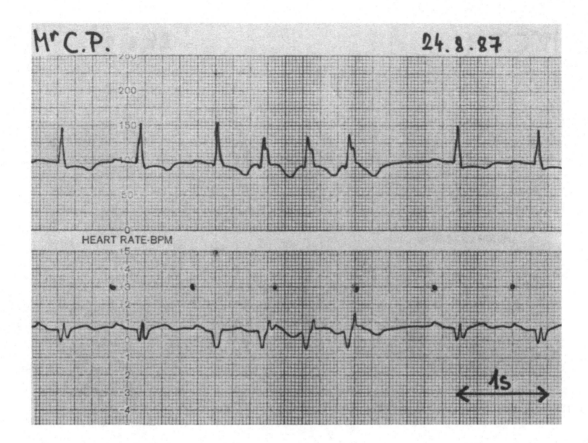

ECG no. 127: Mr. C.P., 75 years

Holter ECG recording

The sinus rhythm with a prolonged PR interval is interrupted by a paroxysmal tachycardia. At first glance, it looks like this paroxysmal tachycardia is composed of three complexes. However, when analyzing the third QRS (•), it becomes clear that it appears slightly earlier after the preceding P wave and that its morphology is very different, especially in the inferior lead. Therefore, this is the first complex of the tachycardia showing fusion with ectopic ventricular activation. The fusion is responsible for a morphology different from that of the QRS during sinus rhythm and the following beats of the tachycardia. Not only is its morphology different, but the duration of the fusion QRS complex is shorter as well. There is a post-tachycardia pause followed by two conducted sinus beats. Note that during ventricular tachycardia, two dissociated sinus P waves are visible (•).

Conclusion

Ventricular tachycardia with fusion of the first beat of tachycardia.

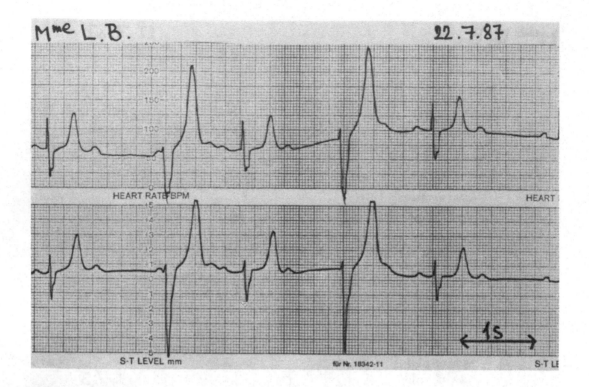

ECG no. 128: Mrs. L.B., 91 years

Malaise
Heart failure
Holter ECG recording

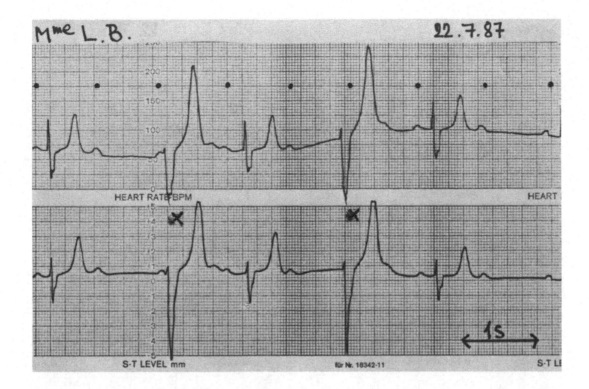

ECG no. 128: Mrs. L.B., 91 years

Holter ECG recording

Sinus rhythm with 2:1 AV block. The first P wave is conducted, resulting in a QRS complex of 140 ms. The second P wave is blocked and followed by a ventricular escape with a wide QRS. The same sequence is repeated thereafter. Note the prolonged PR of the third QRS because of retrograde penetration of the ventricular escape. The conducted beats show QRS widening (140 ms), suggesting bundle branch block. The two leads do not allow us to be more precise about the type of bundle branch block.

Conclusion

2:1 AV block with a ventricular escape rhythm (X).

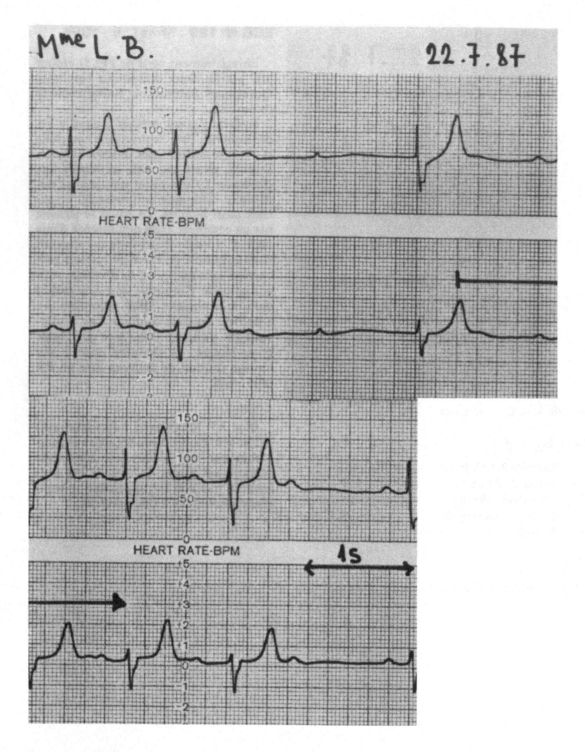

ECG no. 129: Mrs. L.B., 91 years

Malaise
Heart failure
Holter ECG recording
Continuous recording

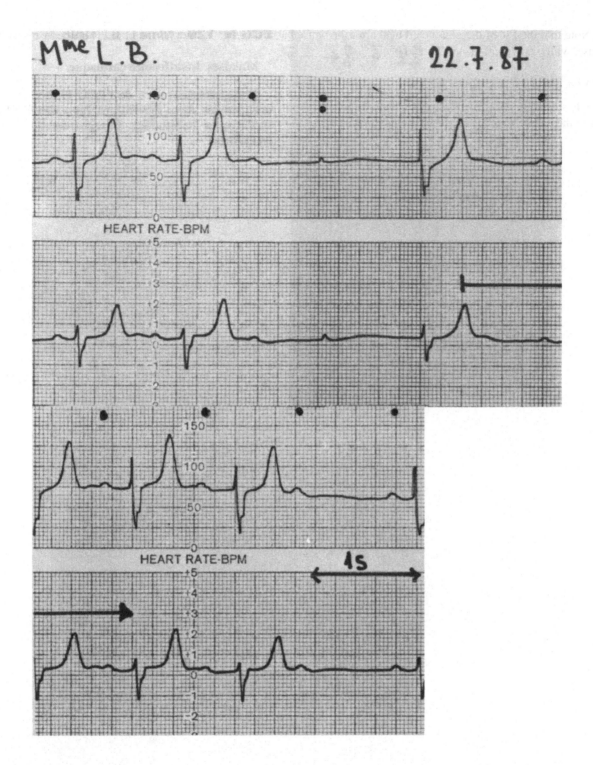

ECG no. 129: Mrs. L.B., 91 years

Holter ECG recording

Continuous recording

   Sinus rhythm with progressive PR prolongation followed by AV block. In the *upper tracing*, the third P wave is blocked. In the pause that follows, there is an ectopic atrial premature beat. The pause is terminated by a QRS complex that is not preceded by a P wave (a junctional escape). The *lower tracing* also shows progressive PR prolongation followed by AV block. Note that the PR of the conducted beat after the pause has a shorter PR interval than the PR of the last beat before the pause, which is typical of AV Wenckebach.

Conclusion

Type 1, second-degree AV block (Wenckebach phenomenon). In the first sequence, there is blocked atrial extrasystole extending the pause, which is ended by a junctional escape.

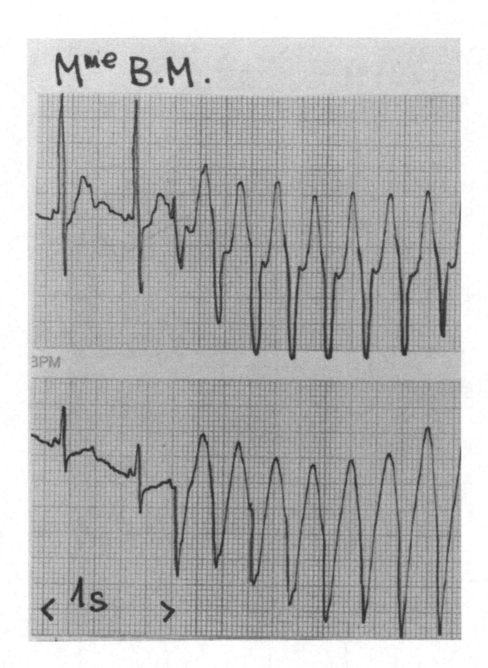

ECG no. 130: Mrs. B.M., 30 years

Palpitations
Vertigo
Holter ECG continuous recording

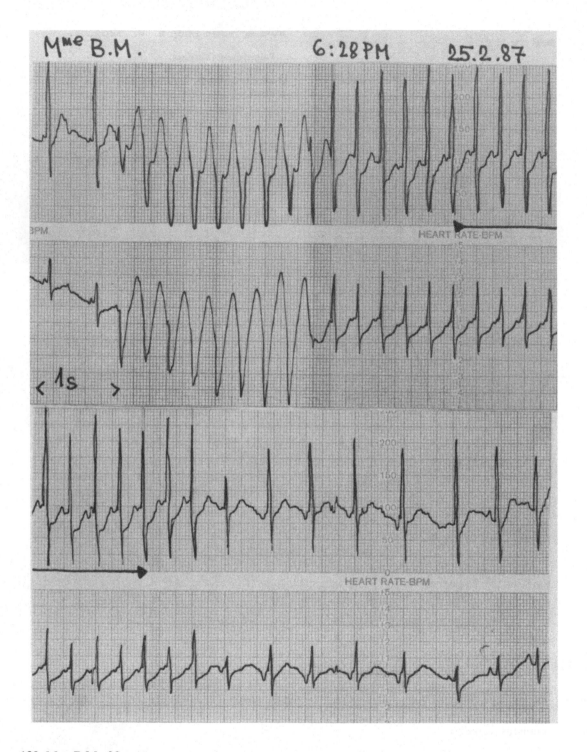

ECG no. 130: Mrs. B.M., 30 years

Holter ECG continuous recording

After two narrow QRS complexes, there is a tachycardia with wide QRS complexes with a QS morphology and a heart rate of 210 bpm. Without a change in tachycardia rate, the ninth and the following 17 QRS complexes have the same morphology as the two QRS complexes at the beginning of the recording. It is difficult to distinguish a P wave during the tachycardia. When the tachycardia stops, we see an accelerated atrial rhythm with a heart rate of 110 bpm and a negative P wave;

after only five complexes of this rhythm, we again see a sinus rhythm. The similar tachycardia rate during the wide and narrow QRS allows the diagnosis of a supraventricular tachycardia. The initial width of the tachycardia may be explained by phase 3 block in the bundle branch, which disappears when the refractory period of the bundle branch shortens during tachycardia. The inability to identify the P wave does not allow a diagnosis to be made regarding the type of supraventricular tachycardia.

Conclusion

Supraventricular tachycardia with an initial phase 3 intraventricular conduction aberration ending with an accelerated atrial rhythm.

NB: If the tachycardia had stopped before the disappearance of the intraventricular conduction aberration or if the recording had stopped too early, a false diagnosis of ventricular tachycardia would have been likely. Therefore, this continuous recording confirms the value of continuous and prolonged monitoring of the arrhythmic events.

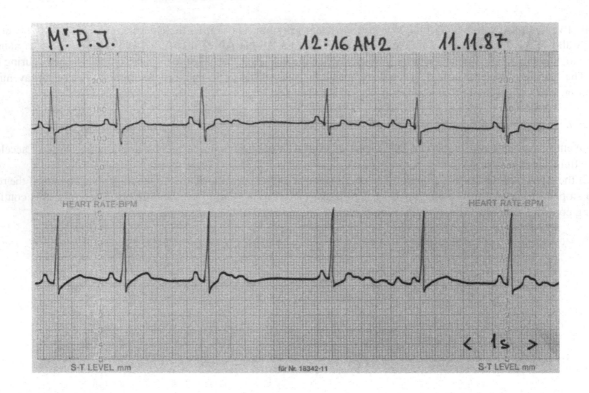

ECG no. 131: Mr. P.J., 33 years

Paroxysmal palpitations
No treatment
Holter ECG recording

68

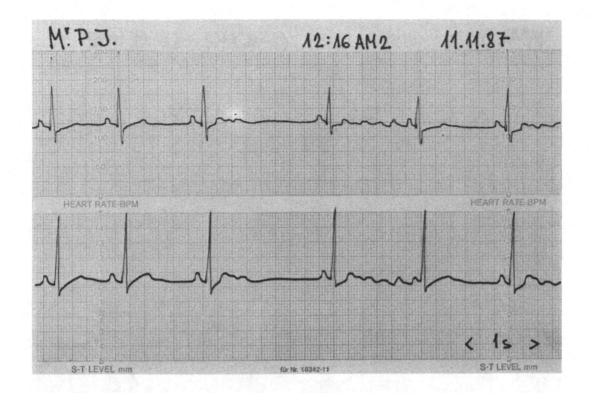

ECG no. 131: Mr. P.J., 33 years

Holter ECG recording

The first three complexes are conducted sinus beats. After the third one, we have rapid ectopic atrial activity in the ST–T segment. This is responsible for a pause because it inactivates the sinus node. We then see a new conducted sinus beat with irregular fast atrial activity in the ST–T segment. One of these atrial events conducts to the ventricle. The same phenomenon of fast atrial activity in the ST–T segment follows the last conducted sinus beat.

Conclusion

Very short onsets of atrial fibrillation. The presence of the pause rules out an artifact.

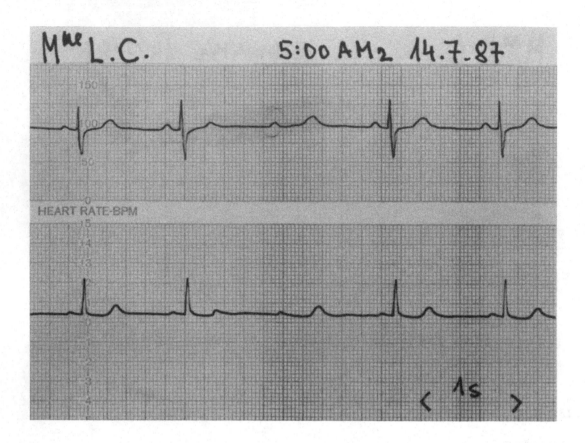

ECG no. 132: Mrs. L.C., 84 years

Heart failure
Angina pectoris
Medication: enalapril, nitroglycerin
Holter ECG recording

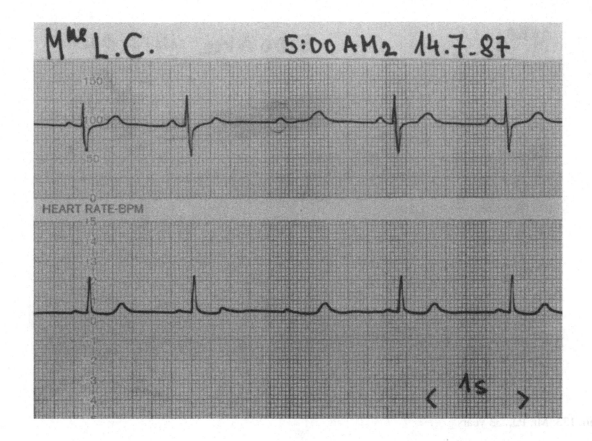

ECG no. 132: Mrs. L.C., 84 years

Holter ECG recording

The sinus rhythm is interrupted by a pause in which we distinguish two waves. The second wave looks like a T wave similar to the one after the first QRS complex. We are in the presence of an artifact that prohibited the inscription of the QRS and also already modified the morphology of the T wave of the second complex. This artifact allowed only the inscription of the P wave and T wave but erased the QRS between.

Conclusion

Artifact.

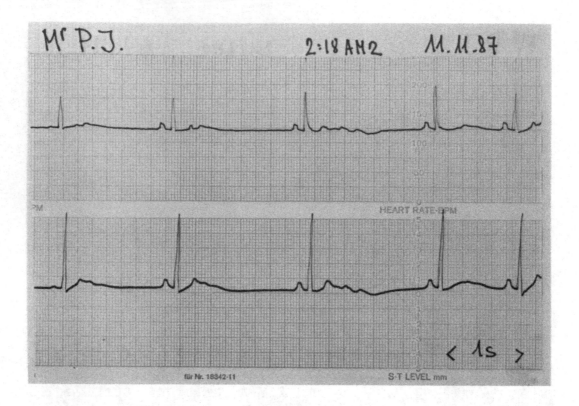

ECG no. 133: Mr. P.J., 33 years

Palpitations
Night recording
Holter ECG recording

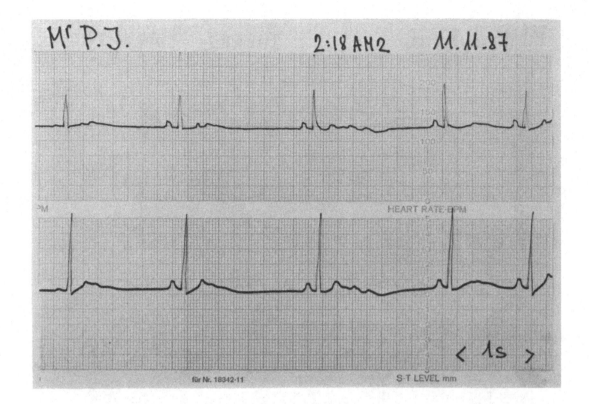

ECG no. 133: Mr. P.J., 33 years

Holter ECG recording

The question whether we are dealing with a real cardiac rhythm or an artifact can possibly be answered by the last two cardiac complexes, which show conducted sinus beats with an R–R interval shorter than those of the previous beats. The rhythm before seems to be altered by ectopic atrial activity in the ST–T segment of the first, second, and third complexes. This activity is seen as one wave after the first QRS, two waves following the second QRS, and three waves after the third QRS. This activity inhibits the sinus activity, decreasing the sinus rate, which is much slower than in the two beats at the end of the tracing, making an artifact unlikely.

Conclusion

Nonconducted ectopic atrial rhythm slowing the sinus rate.

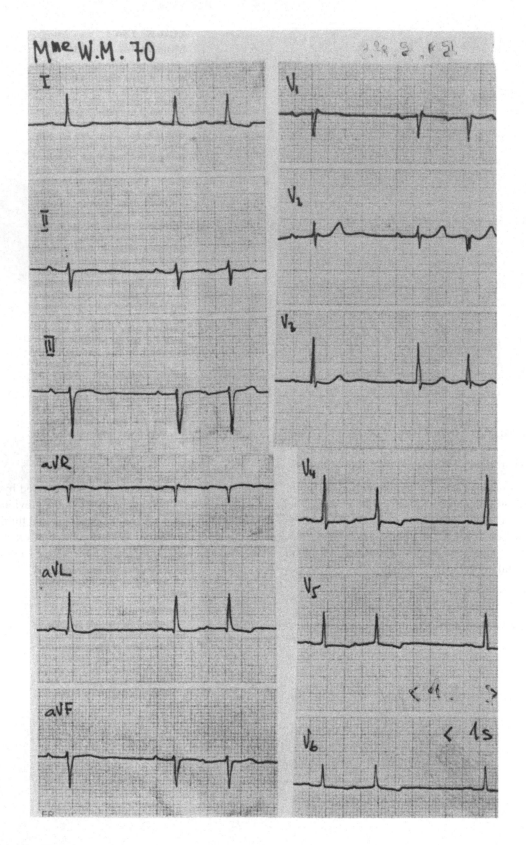

ECG no. 134: Mrs. W.M., 70 years
Vertigo
Malaise
No treatment

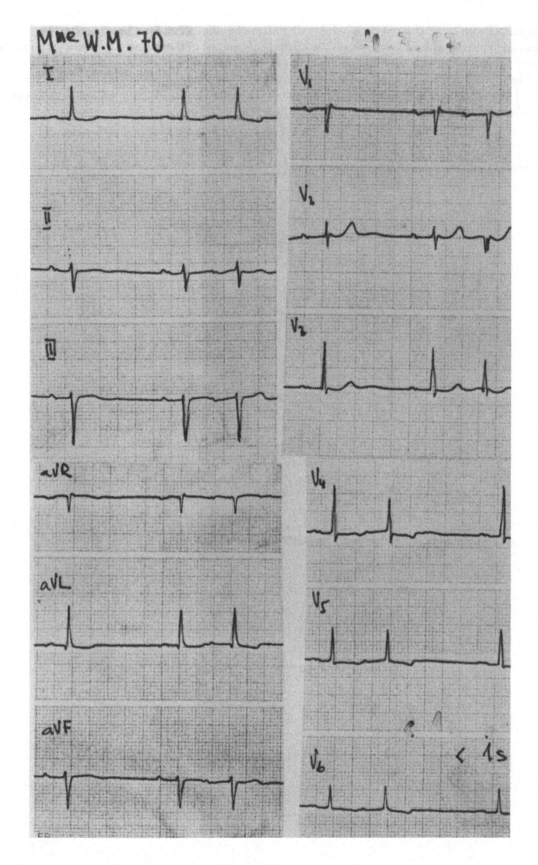

ECG no. 134: Mrs. W.M., 70 years

Sinus bradycardia with coupled atrial extrasystoles. The first two complexes have a heart rate of 47 bpm. The P waves preceding them are biphasic, with a PR interval of 0.26 s. The configuration of the P wave suggests atrial dilatation. The two conducted sinus beats are followed by a different P wave after a shorter interval. The coupling interval is the same in the extremity and the precordial leads. The interval between the ectopic P wave and sinus P wave and the different configuration both exclude 2:1 sinoatrial block as the cause of the bradycardia. Note the further PR prolongation of the coupled atrial premature beat and slight QRS aberrancy after the atrial premature beat.

Conclusion

Sinus bradycardia with coupled atrial premature beats.

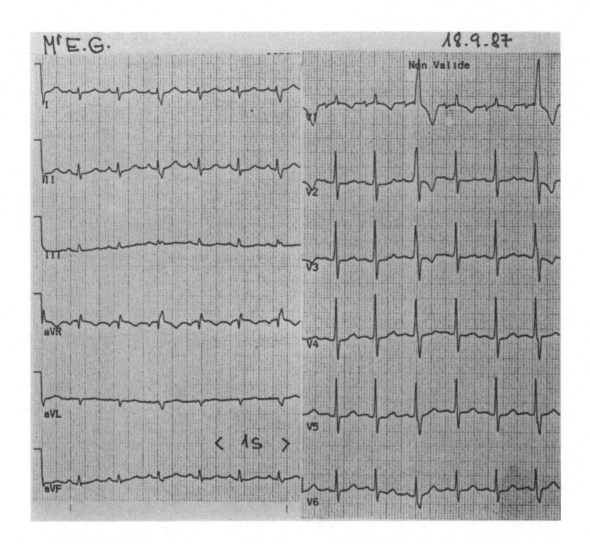

ECG no. 135: Mr. E.G., 60 years

Hypertension
Chronic obstructive pulmonary disease
Medication: digoxin, diuretics

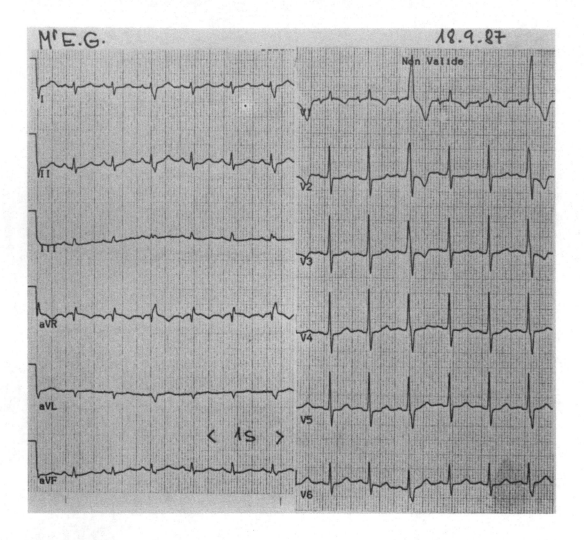

ECG no. 135: Mr. E.G., 60 years

Regular sinus tachycardia of 110 bpm with identical PR intervals. The ventricular complexes have two morphologies:

–   First, we see a QRS complex of 0.10 s with an axis in the frontal plane of 120°, presenting in lead V_1 as an rsR's'.
–   Then we see another QRS complex of 0.13 s with an axis shifted to the right. This QRS has a slightly different appearance in lead V_1, being an rsR', and has a wide S wave in lead V_6. Every third complex presents this second morphologic type.

Conclusion

Incomplete right bundle branch block becoming complete once in three events. The diagnosis is possible because the PR intervals stay identical with both QRS morphologies.

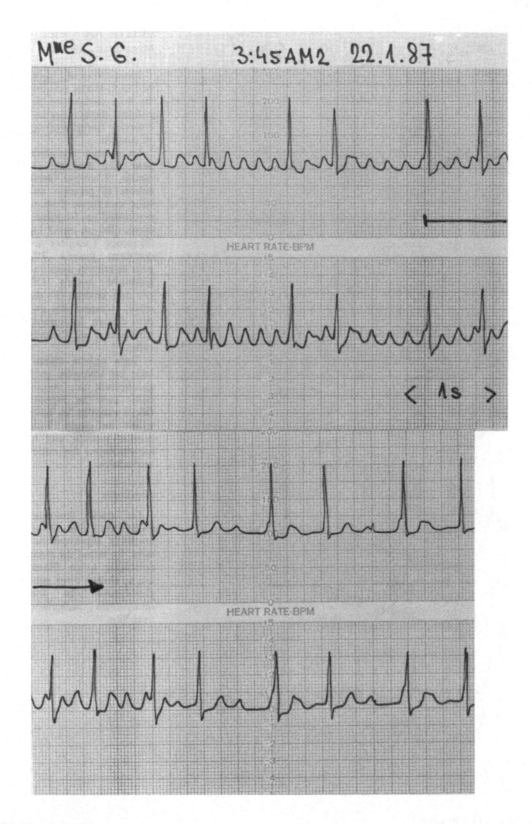

ECG no. 136: Mrs. S.G., 56 years

Palpitations, dyspnea
Continuous Holter ECG recording
Recorded without any symptomatology described by the patient during the night
Medication: digoxin, 1 pill per day

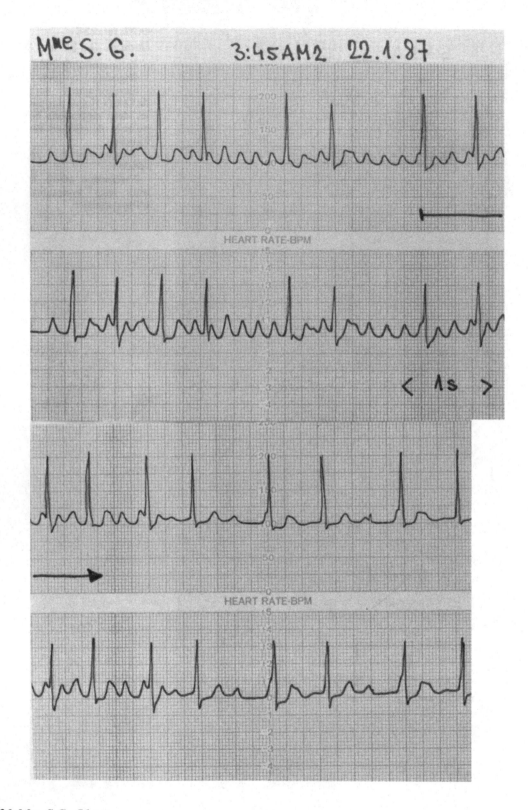

ECG no. 136: Mrs. S.G., 56 years

Continuous Holter ECG recording

The first complex may be of sinus origin. The atrial activity thereafter shows positive waves with an atrial rate of 300 bpm. The frequency accelerates slightly up to 350 bpm followed by marked slowing of the rhythm, with an atrial rate of around

150 bpm at the end of the recording. The morphology of the atrial waves changes, and the amplitude is diminished. This atrial activity is transmitted irregularly to the ventricles with variable block. The QRS morphology is slightly altered by superposition of the atrial waves.

Conclusion

The beginning of the tracing shows atrial flutter with irregular AV conduction, changing into atrial tachycardia with AV block at the end.

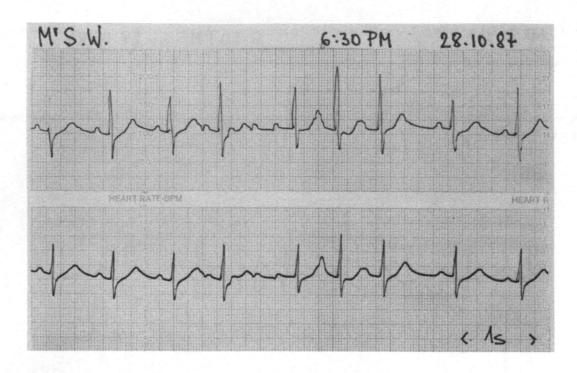

ECG no. 137: Mr. S.W., 70 years

Palpitations
Medication: amiodarone, 1 pill per day 5 days/week
Holter ECG recording
No symptomatology noted by the patient

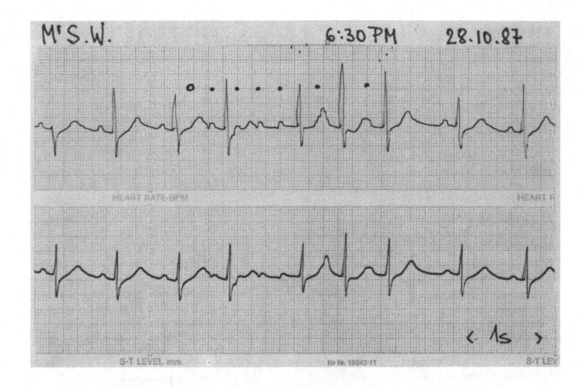

ECG no. 137: Mr. S.W., 70 years

Holter ECG recording

The first three complexes are of sinus origin. Then there is an episode of ectopic atrial rhythm, with an atrial rate of around 180 bpm. This rhythm may be seen at the end of the T wave of the third QRS complex but may be noticed even earlier in the ST segment (○). The ectopic atrial activity (•) is conducted irregularly to the ventricle with identical QRS complexes. The ectopic atrial activity stops abruptly, followed by two conducted sinus beats.

Conclusion

Short episode of atrial tachycardia with AV block; prolonged QT interval during amiodarone treatment.

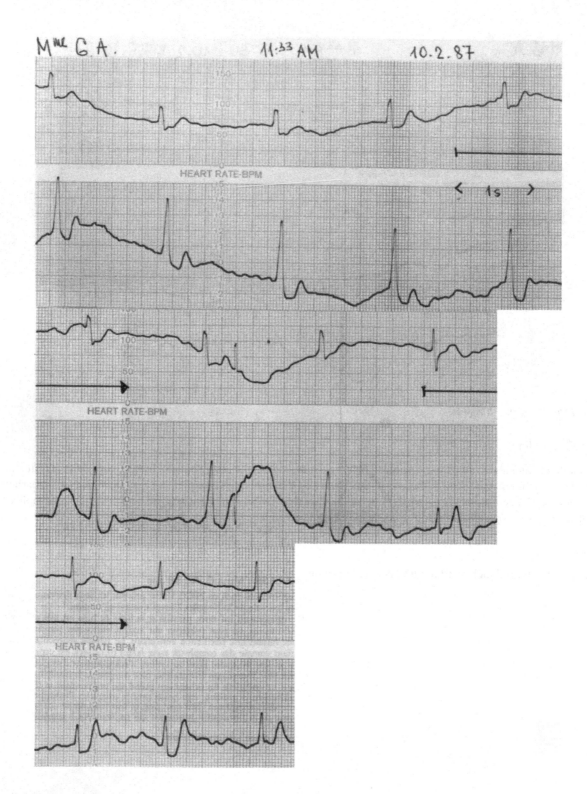

ECG no. 138: Mrs. G.A., 58 years

Heart failure
Dilated cardiomyopathy
Medication: digoxin, 1 pill per day
Continuous Holter ECG recording

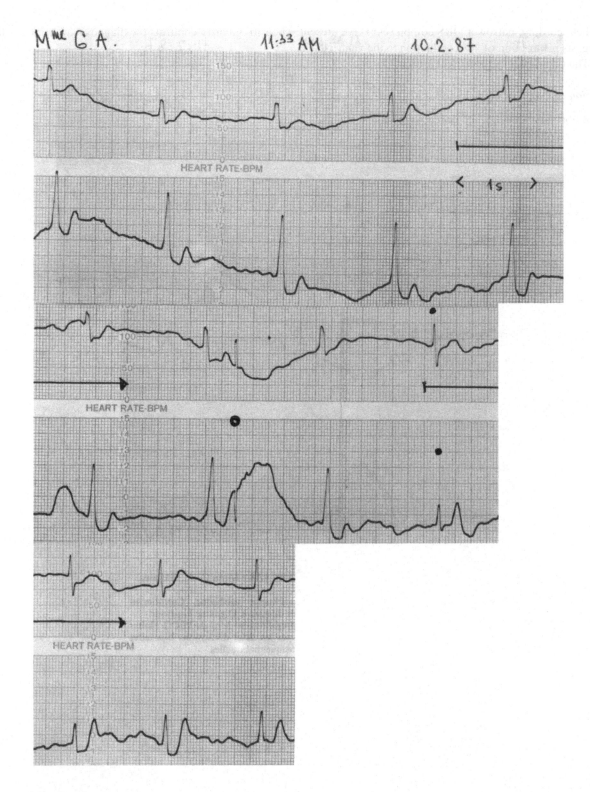

ECG no. 138: Mrs. G.A., 58 years

Continuous Holter ECG recording

Interpretation hampered by the undulating base line. Nevertheless, we recognize rapid atrial activity that is irregular, suggesting atrial fibrillation. The QRS at the beginning of the tracing is wide (0.12 s). The ventricular rhythm is slow and regular, indicating a ventricular escape rhythm (heart rate of 40 bpm) because of complete AV block during atrial fibrillation. At the end of the recording, narrower QRS complexes (•) are present. Their irregularity confirms the diagnosis of atrial fibrillation and suggests resumption of AV conduction to the ventricle.

NB: The (○) mark is an electrical artifact.

Conclusion

Atrial fibrillation with high-degree AV block.

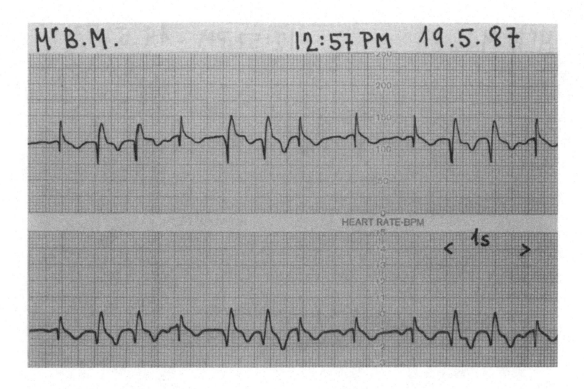

ECG no. 139: Mr. B.M., 37 years

Holter ECG recording
The polarity of the tracing is inverted to facilitate the automatic reading

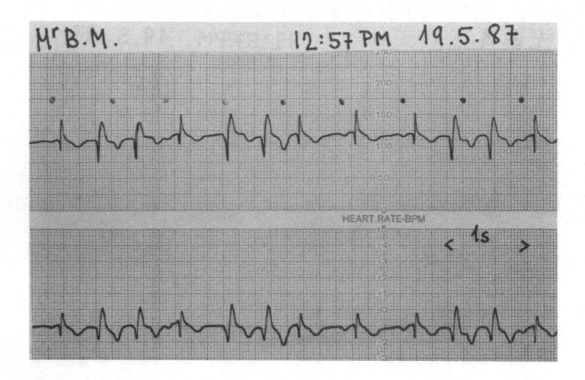

ECG no. 139: Mr. B.M., 37 years

Holter ECG recording

Conducted sinus beats (first, fourth, seventh, eighth, ninth, and eleventh complexes) are interrupted by ventricular complexes wider than the conducted sinus beats. The rhythm of the sinus P waves is regular (•). The wide ventricular complexes are VPBs in doublets without retrograde conduction to the atria but with concealed retrograde conduction, responsible for the lengthening of the PR interval of the sinus complex following the extrasystoles.

NB: The tracing polarity was inverted to facilitate automatic reading, which prefers positive deflections.

Conclusion

Sinus rhythm with frequent VPBs occurring as doublets.

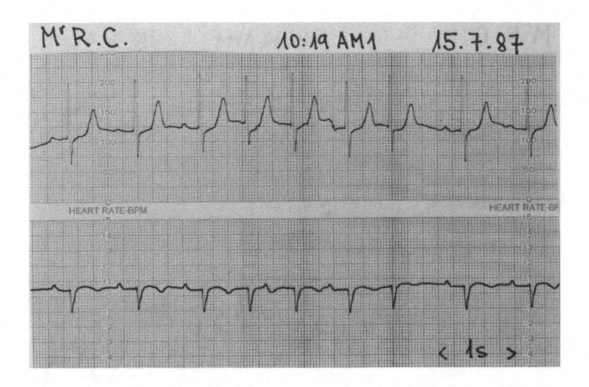

ECG no. 140: Mr. R.C., 52 years

Palpitations
No treatment
Holter ECG recording

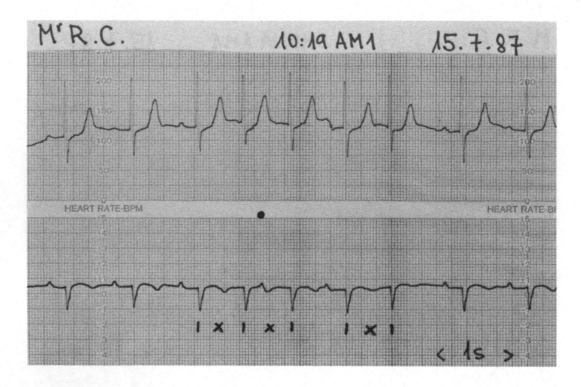

ECG no. 140: Mr. R.C., 52 years

Holter ECG recording

Initially conducted sinus beats with a PR interval of 0.24 s are present. The third P wave is followed by two QRS complexes that are identical. The same sequence is seen following the fifth sinus P wave. These are examples of so-called 1:2 AV conduction, which may occur in the presence of dual AV nodal pathways. The first QRS is the result of AV conduction over a rapidly conducting AV nodal pathway, and the second is the result of AV conduction over a slowly conducting AV nodal pathway. We therefore have two QRS after one P wave! The fourth P wave is followed by a single QRS but with a prolonged PR, indicating retrograde invasion of the fast AV nodal pathway. The last two complexes show sinus beats with 1:1 conduction to the ventricle.

Conclusion

Example of 1:2 AV conduction during sinus rhythm in the presence of dual AV nodal pathways.

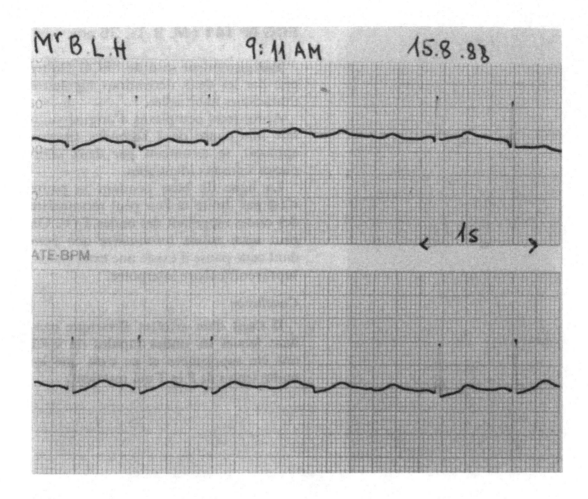

ECG no. 141: Mr. B.L., 35 years

Palpitations
No treatment
Holter ECG recording

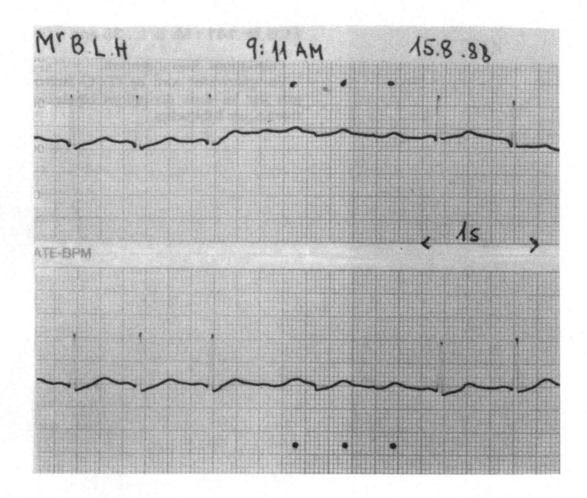

ECG no. 141: Mr. B.L., 35 years

Holter ECG recording

The first three complexes are conducted sinus beats. Thereafter, there is a 2-s pause without a QRS that terminates with two conducted sinus beats. The baseline during the pause is not straight, and we can recognize some waves that remind us of T waves (•). These apparent T waves suggest that during this pause, an interpolated supraventricular extrasystole is present.

Conclusion

This is an electrical artifact. During the recording, the fast QRS waves were suppressed, and we see only the T waves that remain.

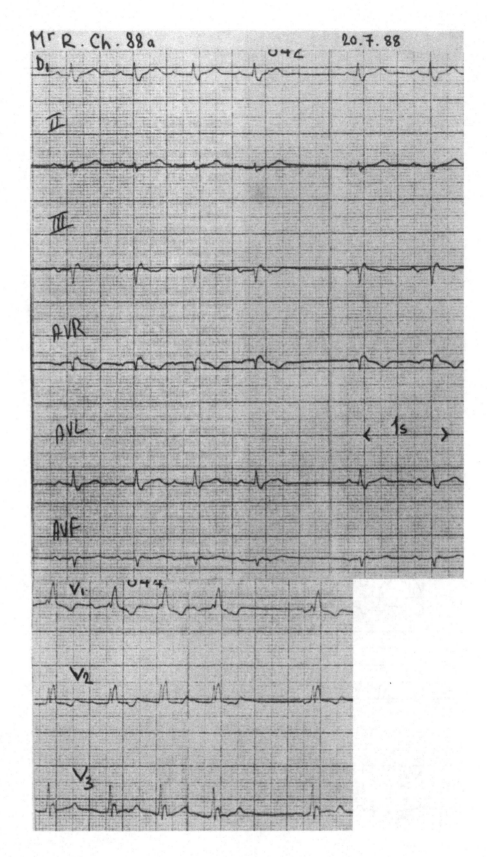

ECG no. 142: Mr. R.Ch., 88 years

Heart failure
Digoxin, 1 pill per day 5 days/week

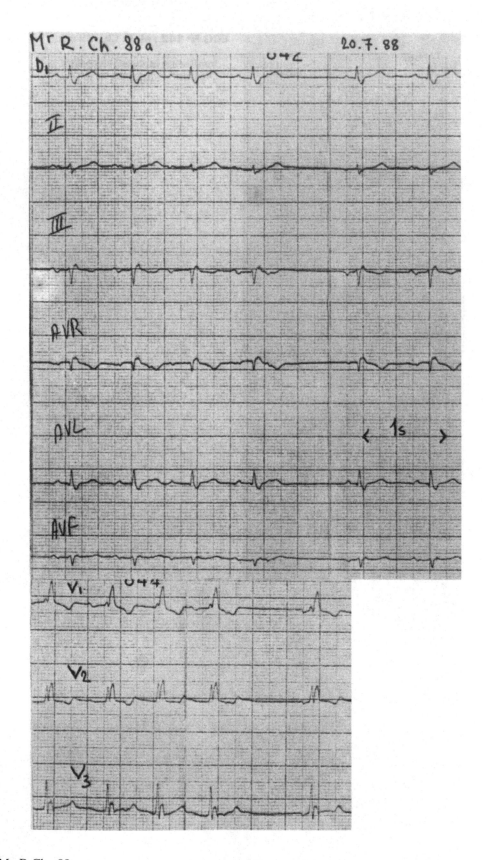

ECG no. 142: Mr. R.Ch., 88 years

Peripheral leads: The first two complexes are conducted sinus beats with a PR interval of 0.22 s and a QRS width of 0.12 s with right bundle branch block. In the T wave after the second QRS complex, there is an ectopic P′ wave followed by a

94

second ectopic P' wave that conducts to the ventricles with an extended PR interval of 0.26 s. The morphology of the ventricular QRS complex is identical to the previous complex. The fourth complex also is of sinus origin; in its T wave, there is a new ectopic P' wave that is not conducted to the ventricle and is followed by a pause that terminates with a P wave, slightly different morphologically (isoelectrical in lead II and negative in lead III), conducting to the ventricles with a shortened PR interval of 0.14 s.

Precordial leads: The first two complexes are conducted sinus beats, and the QRS morphology shows a complete right bundle branch block. In the beginning of the T wave of the second complex, there is an ectopic P' wave, seen especially clearly in lead V_3, which is conducted to the ventricle with a markedly prolonged PR interval of 0.36 s. The next conducted sinus complex has a slightly extended PR interval. In its ST segment, we again see a new ectopic P' wave, which is blocked, inducing a pause, terminated with a P wave different from the sinus P wave, and conducted to the ventricle with a shortened PR interval of 0.14 s, suggesting a low atrial escape beat like the one following the pause in the extremity lead recording.

Conclusion

Increased ectopic atrial excitability blocked or conducted to the ventricle. The pauses terminate with a low atrial escape.

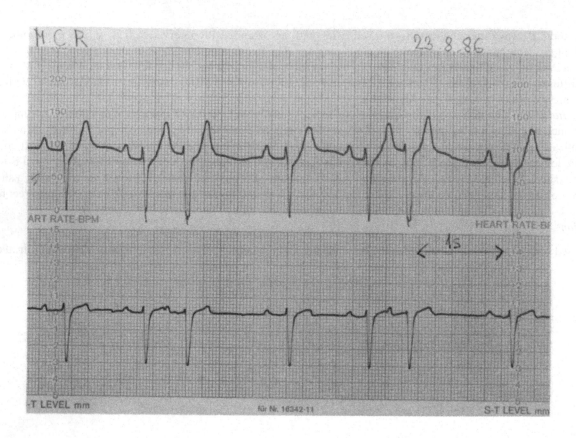

ECG no. 143: Mr. C.R., 64 years

Aortic stenosis
Palpitations
No medication
Holter ECG recording

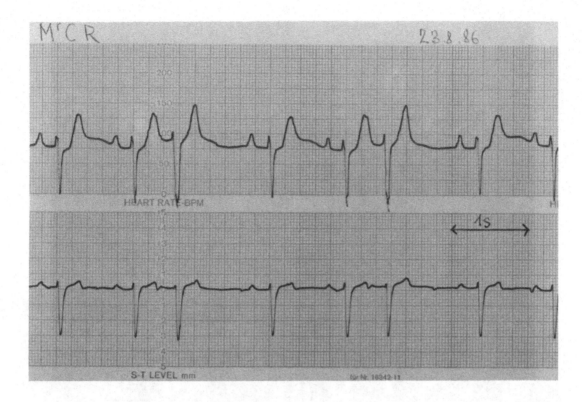

ECG no. 143: Mr. C.R., 64 years

Holter ECG recording

Conducted sinus rhythm with a PR interval of 0.28 s (first two complexes) is interrupted by atrial premature beats with a QRS similar to that of the conducted sinus beat but a little longer (0.12 s). The widening of the QRS complex is the result of intraventricular conduction aberration.

Conclusion

Sinus rhythm with coupled atrial premature beats.

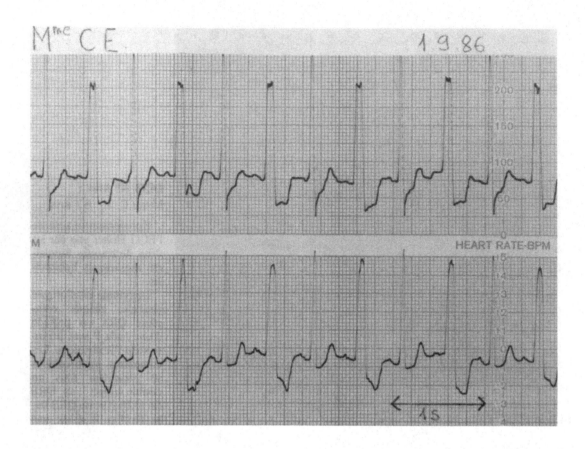

ECG no. 144: Mrs. C.E., 67 years

Palpitations
Shortness of breath on exercise
Malaise during exercise
Holter ECG recording

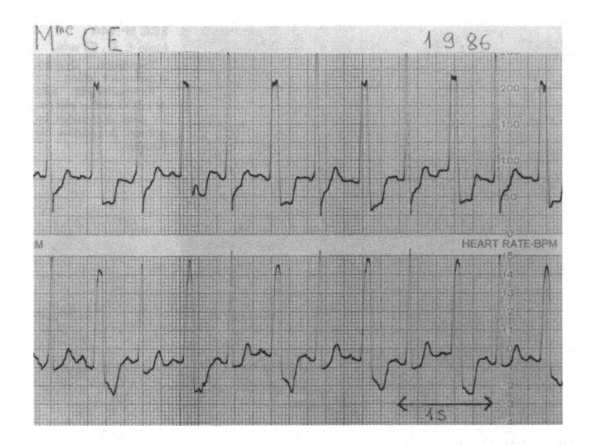

ECG no. 144: Mrs. C.E., 67 years

Holter ECG recording

Sinus tachycardia. Each QRS complex is preceded by a P wave with an identical PR interval. The ventricular complexes present a double morphology: one is a narrow QRS (0.10 s), and the other is a wide QRS (0.14 s). The alternating QRS configuration may be explained by 2:1 block in the bundle branch.

Conclusion

Sinus tachycardia with 2:1 bundle branch block.

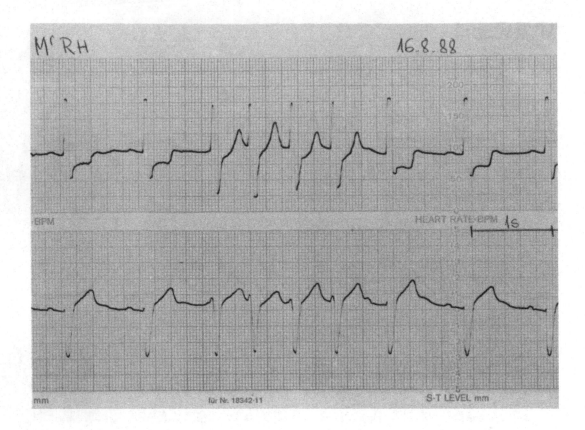

ECG no. 145: Mr. R.H., 62 years

History of myocardial infarction
Holter ECG recording
Asymptomatic patient during recording

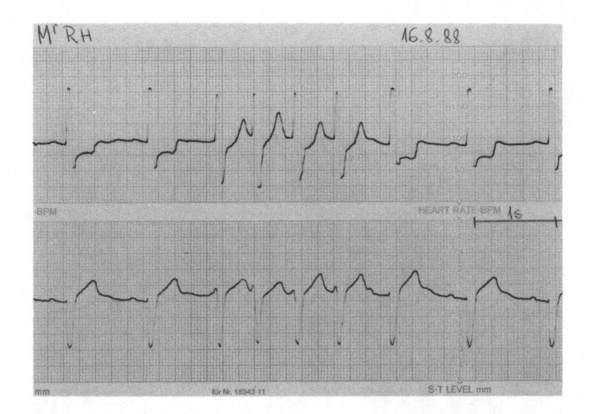

ECG no. 145: Mr. R.H., 62 years

Holter ECG recording

The first two complexes are conducted sinus beats with a wide QRS of 0.16 s and clear ST segment deviation. Thereafter, a tachycardia of four QRS complexes occurs with a heart rate of 120 bpm. The presence of AV dissociation and the fact that the QRS and the ST–T segment during tachycardia are clearly different from the conducted QRS–T complex indicate that a ventricular tachycardia is present. The AV conduction of the first sinus P wave following the tachycardia is lengthened because of retrograde concealed conduction of the last ventricular tachycardia beat.

Conclusion

Ventricular tachycardia.

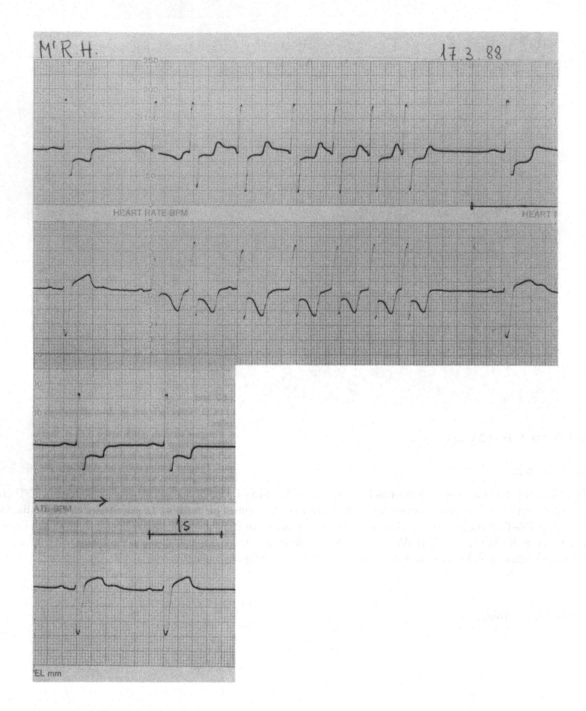

ECG no. 146: Mr. R.H., 62 years

History of myocardial infarction
Holter ECG recording
Asymptomatic patient during recording

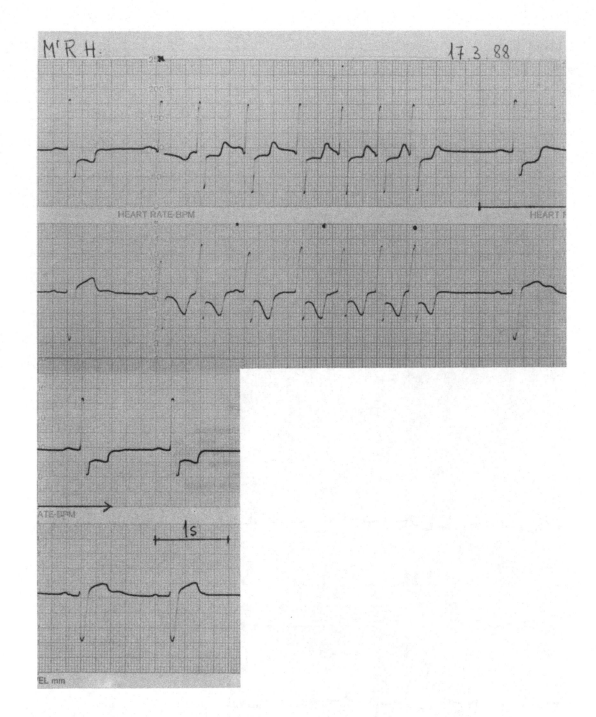

ECG no 146: Mr. R.H., 62 years

Holter ECG recording

The first QRS complex is of sinus origin (QRS duration of 0.12 s). Thereafter, a wide QRS tachycardia (0.16 s) occurs with gradual rate acceleration, from 100 to 125 bpm. The ventricular origin of the tachycardia is confirmed by the AV dissociation; the sinus P waves may be followed during the whole tachycardic event (•). We also note a fusion phenomenon in the first complex of the tachycardia (X) between the tachycardia beat and the conducted sinus P wave.

Conclusion

Ventricular tachycardia.

103

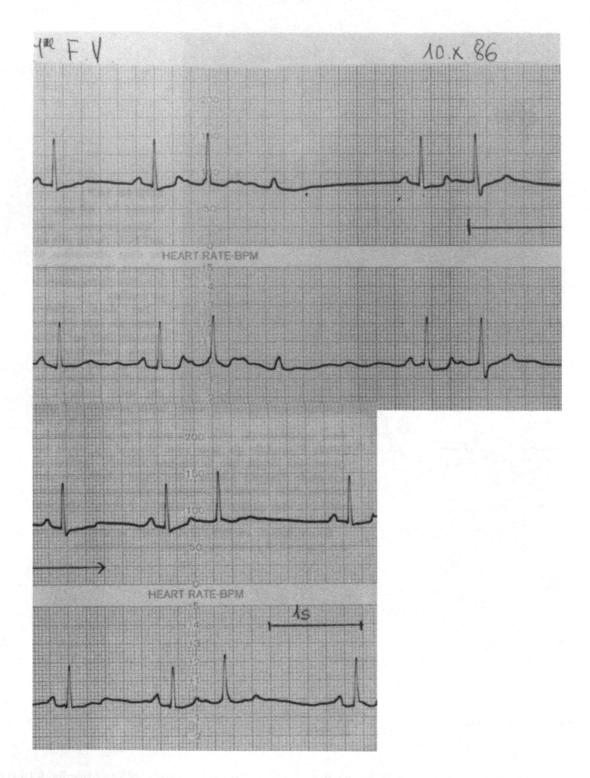

ECG no. 147: Mrs. F.V., 47 years

Palpitations
No treatment
Continuous Holter ECG recording

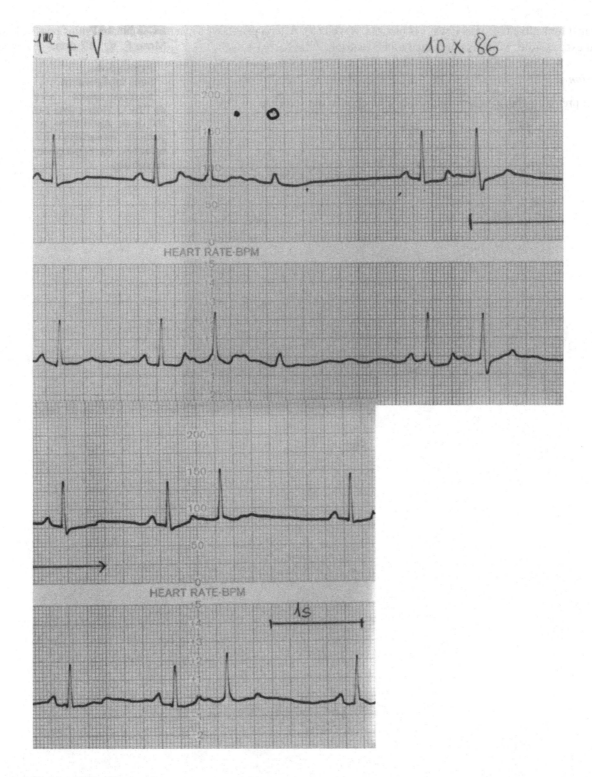

ECG no. 147: Mrs. F.V., 47 years

Continuous Holter ECG recording

The first two complexes are conducted sinus beats. We then see a conducted premature atrial extrasystole and a new ectopic P' wave hidden in the T wave of this extrasystole. This last ectopic P' wave is not conducted to the ventricle (•). A new

105

P wave that looks like the sinus P wave is blocked as well (○). After a pause, we see a new conducted sinus beat followed by an atrial extrasystole, which is conducted to the ventricle.

Conclusion

Atrial premature beats either conducted or blocked to the ventricle.

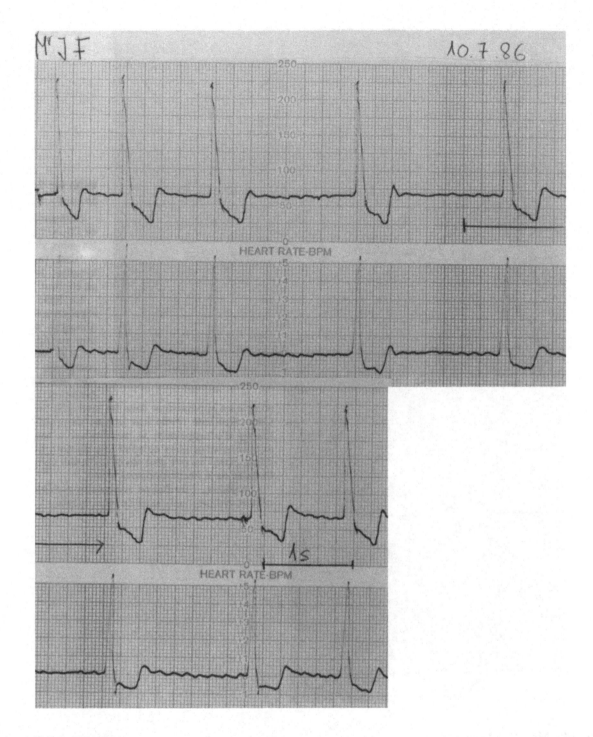

ECG no. 148: Mr. J.F., 82 years

Palpitations
Malaise
Continuous Holter ECG recording

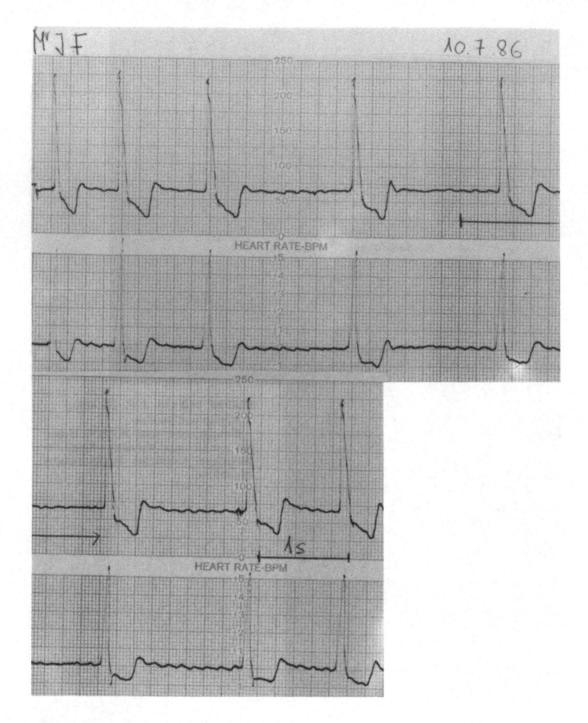

ECG no. 148: Mr. J.F., 82 years

Continuous Holter ECG recording

The baseline is completely irregular, indicating atrial fibrillation. When the R–R intervals are measured, it becomes clear that the long intervals are identical. This indicates that a high degree of AV block is present with episodes of complete AV block terminated by AV junctional escapes.

Conclusion

Atrial fibrillation with episodes of complete AV block and escapes.

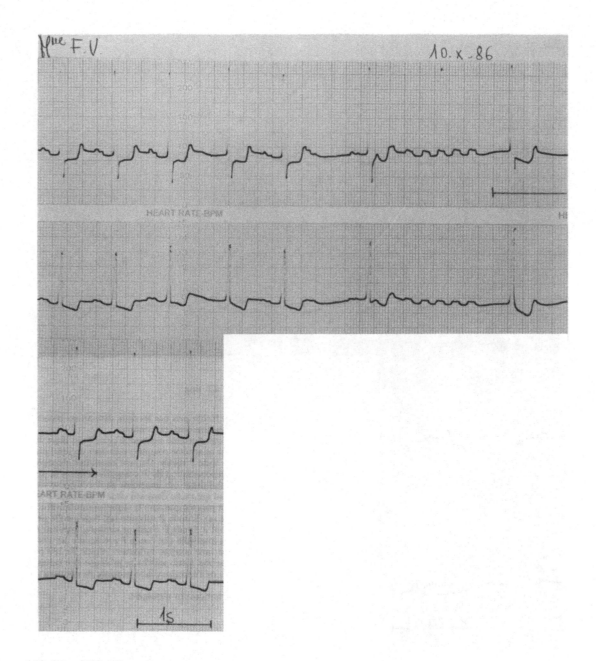

ECG no. 149: Mrs. F.V., 47 years

Palpitations
Shortness of breath
Continuous Holter ECG monitoring

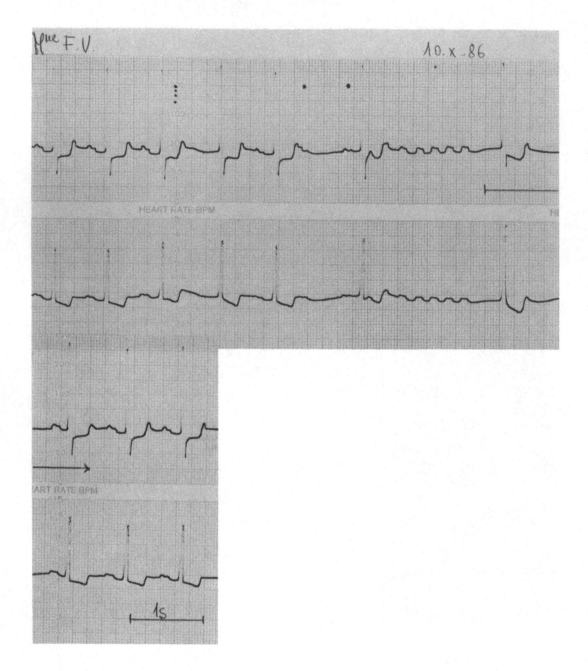

ECG no. 149: Mrs. F.V., 47 years

Continuous Holter ECG monitoring

The first three complexes are of sinus origin. The P wave is wide and biphasic, and the PR interval is 0.26 s. The fourth QRS complex follows after a delay. At first sight, no P wave seems to precede this complex. However, there is a notch in the repolarization phase of the third complex, indicating an ectopic P′ wave conducted with delay to the fourth ventricular complex (■). A conducted sinus beat follows, again with a blocked P′ wave in its T wave (•). After the pause, another conducted sinus P is seen. Starting in the QRS, monomorphic atrial activity of 280 bpm may be observed. That episode is terminated by a junctional escape. The last three complexes of the tracing represent conducted sinus rhythm.

Conclusion

Intermittent atrial hyperexcitability with a possible sequence of short-duration atrial flutter.

110

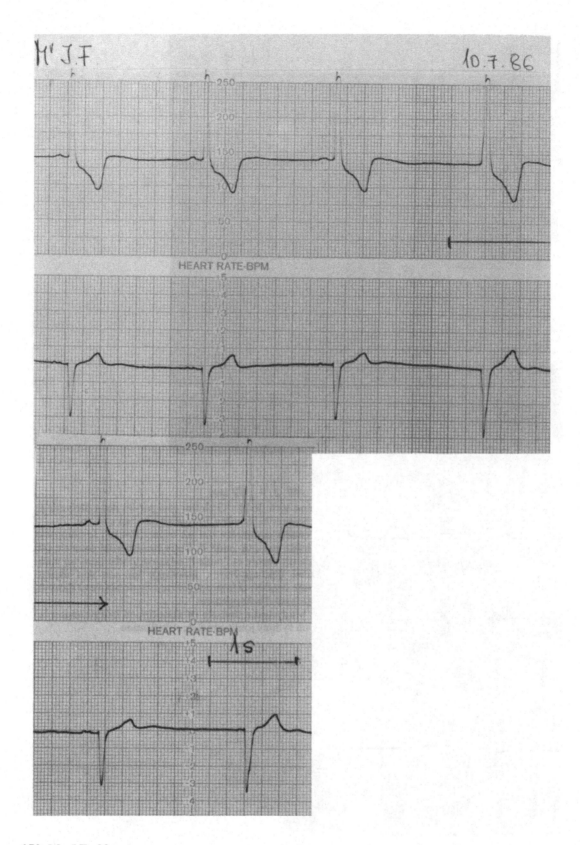

ECG no. 150: Mr. J.F., 82 years

Palpitations
Malaise
Continuous Holter ECG recording

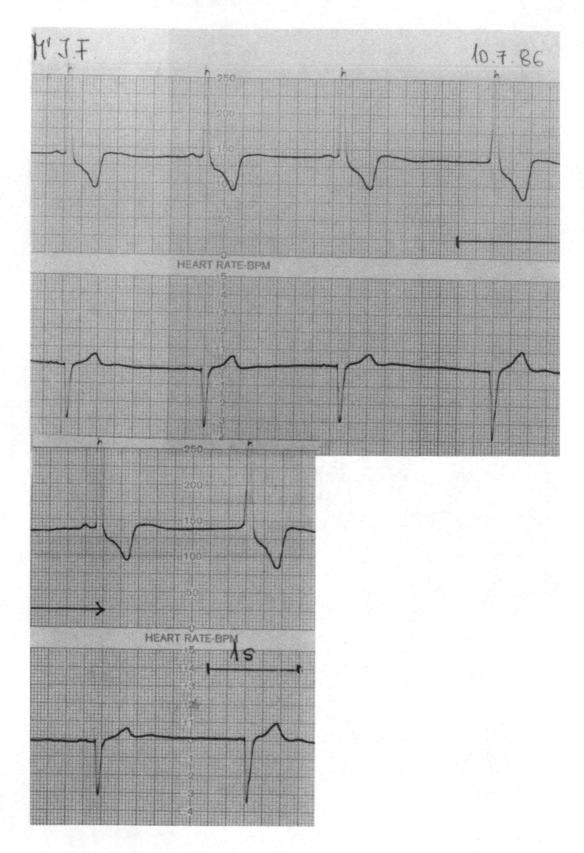

ECG no. 150: Mr. J.F., 82 years

Continuous Holter ECG recording

Severe sinus bradycardia with normal AV conduction (PR, 160 ms) to the ventricle and AV junctional escapes (beats 4 and 6)

Conclusion

Sinus bradycardia with a junctional escape rhythm.

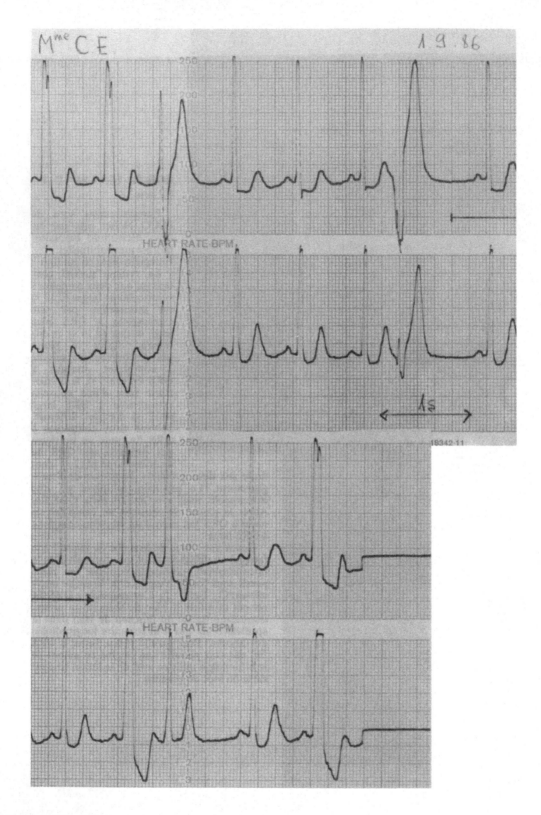

ECG no. 151: Mrs. C.E., 67 years

Palpitations
Shortness of breath
Malaise on exercise
Continuous Holter ECG recording

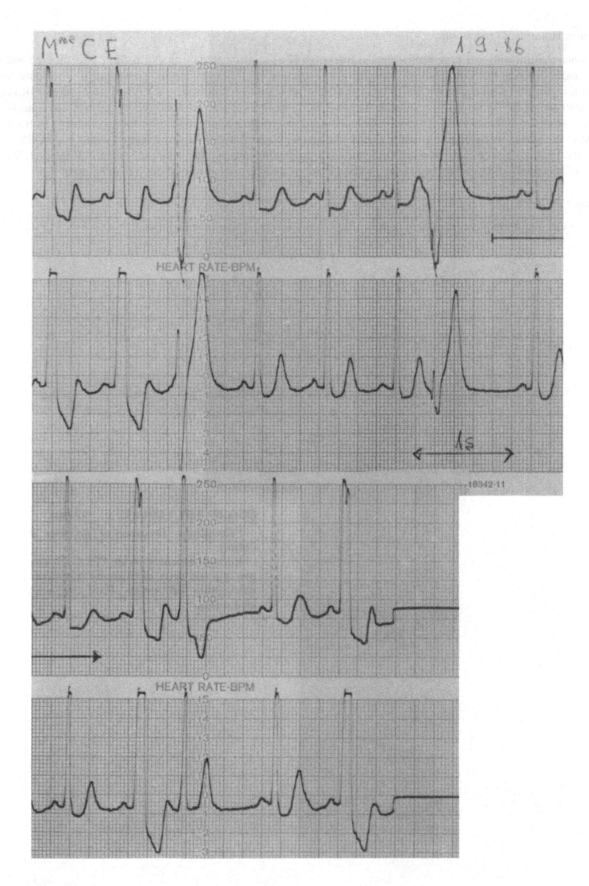

ECG no. 151: Mrs. C.E., 67 years

Continuous Holter ECG recording

The sinus rhythm with two wide ventricular complexes (0.12 s) is interrupted by an extrasystole with an even wider QRS (0.16 s) and a different QRS morphology, indicating a ventricular origin. Following the post-extrasystolic pause, we have three sinus complexes with a narrow QRS (0.08 s), the last of which is also followed by a VPB with a different QRS configuration. After the pause, we have two conducted narrow QRS complexes. These are followed by a conducted sinus beat with a wide QRS (0.12 s) identical to the first two complexes of the recording. The next QRS is an extrasystole but with a narrower QRS. After the pause, we again find two sinus QRS, the first with a narrow QRS and the second with a wide QRS complex. Repeatedly, it may be seen that the wide QRS during sinus rhythm occurs after a shorter sinus P–P interval. This is an example of acceleration-dependent bundle branch block occurring after a sinus rate of more than 85 bpm.

Conclusion

Sinus rhythm with frequent premature beats and acceleration-related bundle branch block.

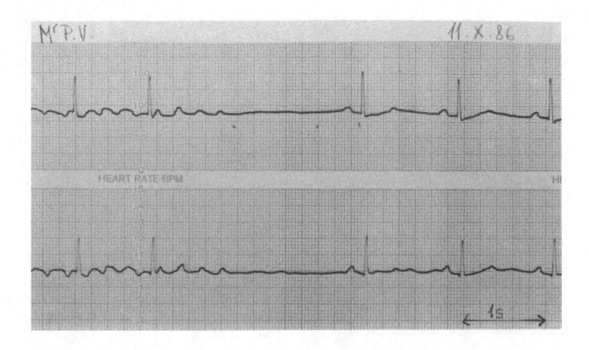

ECG no. 152: Mr. P.V., 47 years

Palpitations
No treatment
Holter ECG monitoring

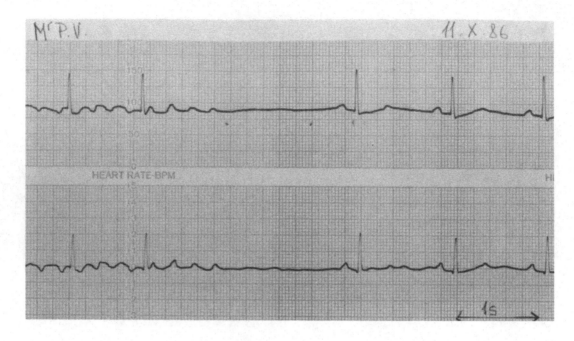

ECG no. 152: Mr. P.V., 47 years

Holter ECG monitoring

The baseline at the beginning of the recording shows a fast irregular atrial rhythm, indicating atrial fibrillation. During atrial fibrillation, two conducted QRS occur. When atrial fibrillation stops, there is a pause of 1.56 s terminated by a conducted sinus P wave. The interval between the next two sinus P waves measures 1.16 s. The duration of the pause is different at the ventricular level (the distance between the two QRS complexes is 2.6 s) and the atrial level (the distance between the last f wave from the atrial fibrillation and the first P wave of sinus origin is only 1.56 s). This allows us to determine the corrected sinus node recovery time by subtracting 1.16 s from 1.56 s, which is 400 ms. This value is below the upper limit of normal for the corrected sinus recovery time of 520 ms, indicating that a sick sinus syndrome in this patient is very unlikely.

Conclusion

Self-terminating episode of atrial fibrillation.

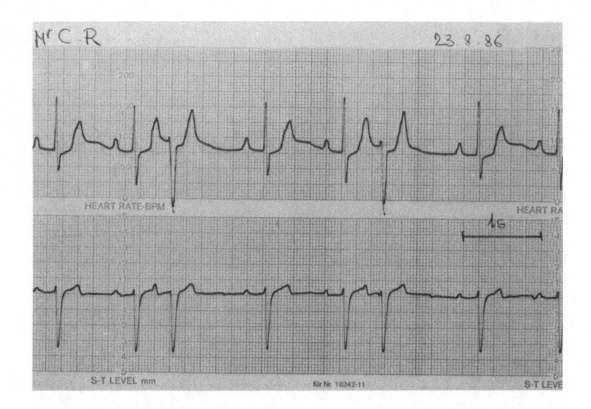

ECG no. 153: Mr. C.R.

Palpitations
Holter ECG monitoring

119

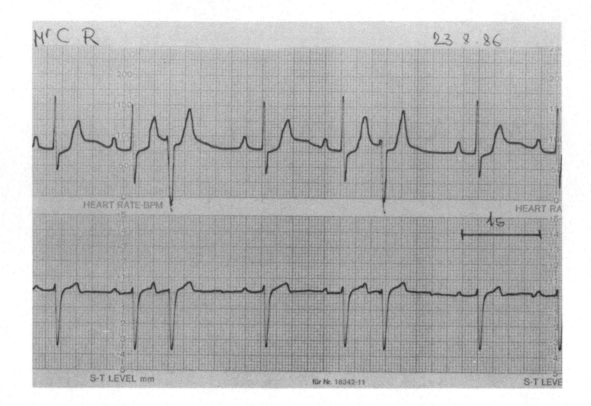

ECG no. 153: Mr. C.R.

Holter ECG monitoring

Sinus rhythm is interrupted by a premature beat inducing a trigeminy. The origin of this premature beat is atrial because we very clearly see the ectopic P′ wave. The ventricular complex has a different configuration and width because of aberrant intraventricular conduction.

Conclusion

Atrial trigeminy with aberrant intraventricular conduction.

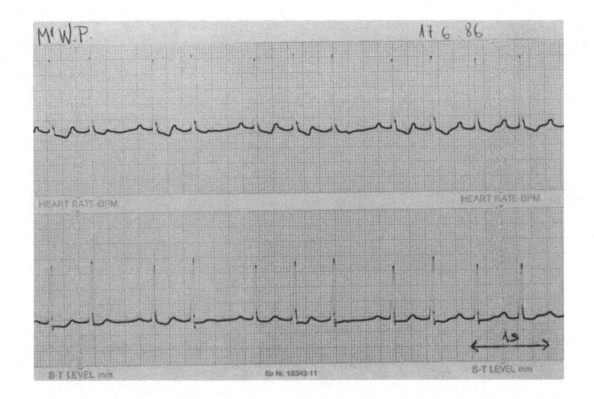

ECG no. 154: Mr. W.P., 49 years

Palpitations
Chest pain
No medication
Holter ECG monitoring

121

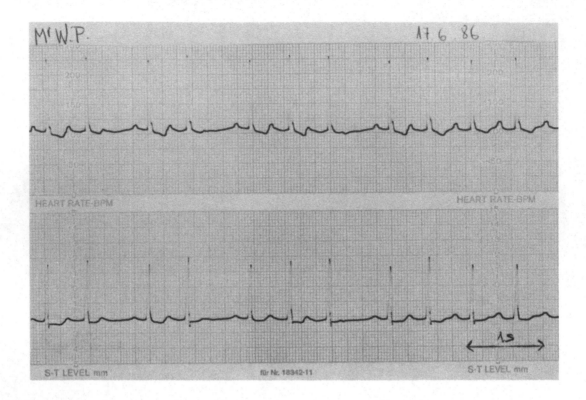

ECG no. 154: Mr. W.P., 49 years

Holter ECG monitoring

The first atrial complex originating in the sinus node is followed by an atrial premature beat. The same sequence occurs after the second sinus beat. The third sinus beat is followed by two premature supraventricular beats, and a paroxysmal atrial tachycardia with a rate of 110 bpm starts at the end of the tracing after the fourth sinus beat.

Conclusion

Frequent ectopic atrial beats followed by paroxysmal atrial tachycardia.

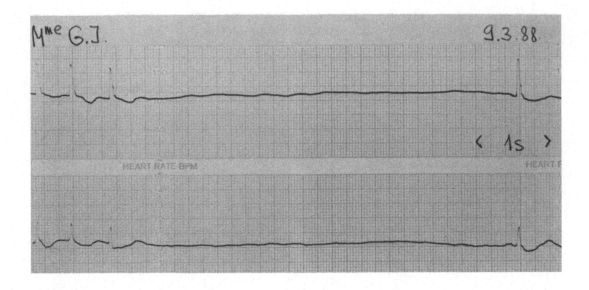

ECG no. 155: Mrs. G.J., 72 years

Malaise
Palpitations
Syncope
No treatment
Holter ECG monitoring

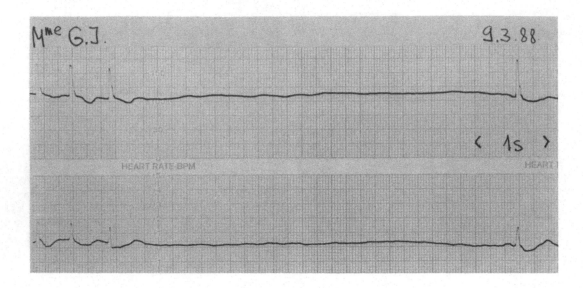

ECG no. 155: Mrs. G.J., 72 years

Holter ECG monitoring

The first three ventricular complexes occur during atrial fibrillation. Then, there is a 5.5-s atrial standstill terminated by a sinus P wave, which is conducted to the ventricle.

Conclusion

An episode of sinus arrest of more than 5 s following the termination of atrial fibrillation indicates sinoatrial disease and is a clear indication for permanent pacing.

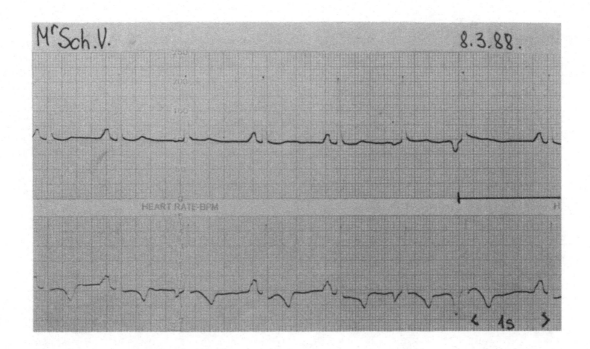

ECG no. 156: Mr. Sch.V., 56 years

Coronary artery disease
Chronic obstructive pulmonary disease
Palpitations
Continuous Holter ECG monitoring

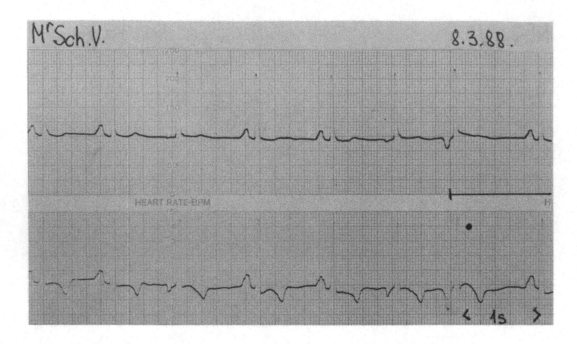

ECG no. 156: Mr. Sch.V., 56 years

Continuous Holter ECG monitoring

The first two ventricular complexes are conducted sinus beats with a PR interval of 0.20 s. The third complex has an identical QRS but arrives slightly earlier and is preceded by a P′ wave with a morphology very different from that of the sinus P wave. The next two complexes are the same as the first two. Then, we have a complex quite similar to the third complex; it is also slightly more premature. The next complex (the seventh from the start of the recording) once again is premature and this time preceded by a P′ wave that is clearly negative in polarity, with a shorter PR interval of 0.13 s. The last complex appears delayed and is of sinus origin. The morphology of the different P waves suggests the possibility in the third and sixth P waves of a fusion between the sinus P wave and the low atrial P wave preceding the seventh QRS. This also explains the slight prematurity of the third and sixth P waves. The seventh P wave represents the low atrial premature beat not modified by any fusion.

Conclusion

Fusion between sinus rhythm and a low atrial rhythm.

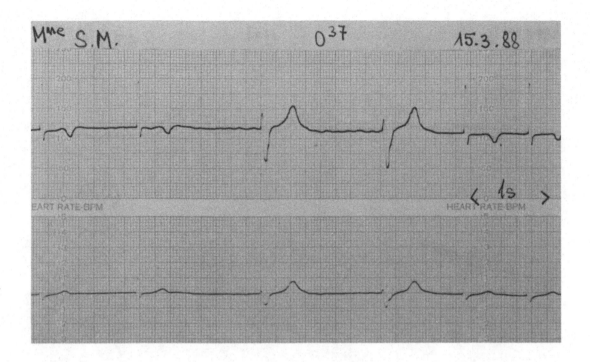

ECG no. 157: Mrs. S.M., 70 years

Palpitations
Vertigo
Malaise
No treatment
Holter ECG monitoring at 00h37
No symptomatology; the patient was asleep

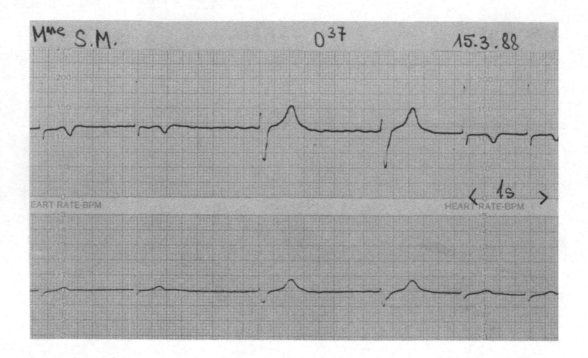

ECG no. 157: Mrs. S.M., 70 years

Holter ECG monitoring

Atrial fibrillation is the arrhythmia at the supraventricular level. The first two (narrow) QRS complexes are conducted over the AV conduction system. Thereafter, two wide QRS complexes are seen after a long, identical R–R interval. This indicates we are dealing with ventricular escapes because of a transitory AV block, which is complete. The last two (narrow) QRS complexes are the result of resumption of AV conduction during atrial fibrillation.

Conclusion

Atrial fibrillation with intermittent complete AV block.

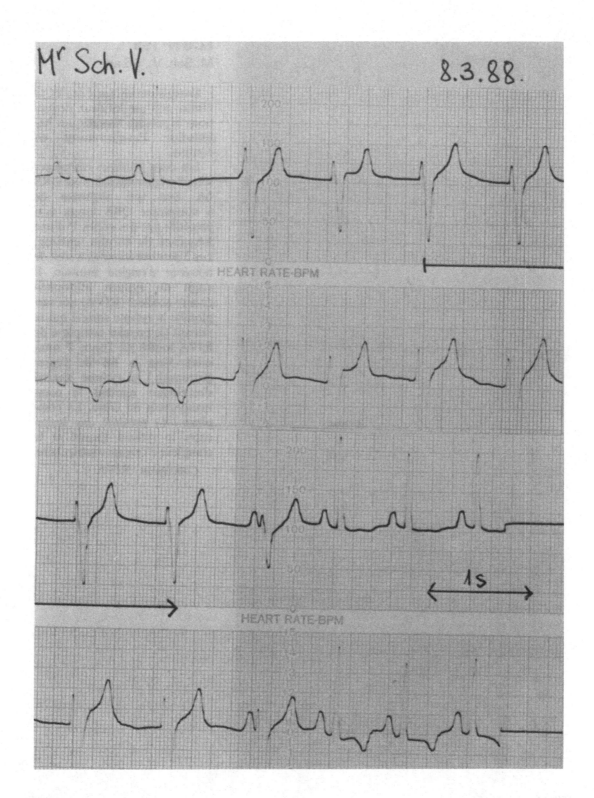

ECG no. 158: Mr. Sch.V., 56 years

Coronary artery disease
Chronic obstructive pulmonary disease
Palpitations
Continuous Holter ECG monitoring

129

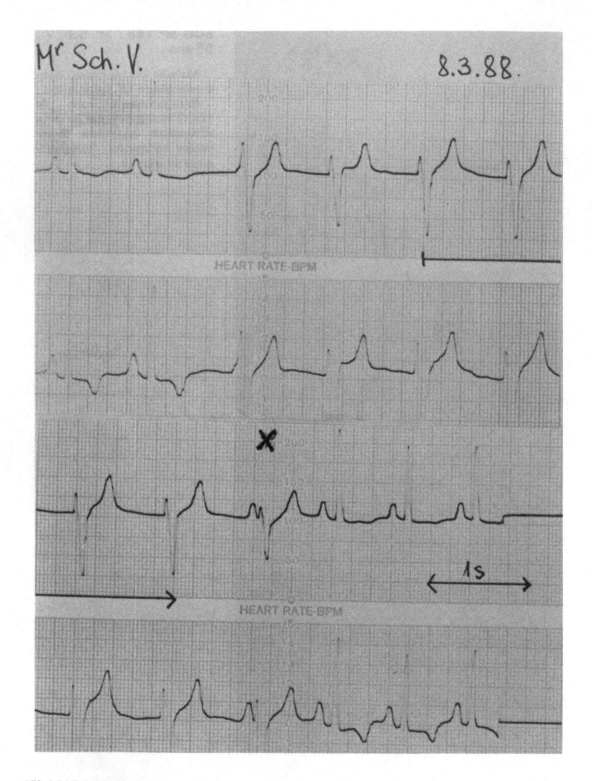

ECG no. 158: Mr. Sch.V., 56 years

Continuous Holter ECG monitoring

The first two complexes are of sinus origin and have a narrow QRS complex. They are followed by six wide QRS complexes not preceded by a P wave, with a heart rate of 66 bpm. The last three complexes also are of sinus origin. The six wide

QRS complexes represent an accelerated idioventricular rhythm (AIVR). This rhythm appears because the sinus rhythm slows down (the first complex of the AIVR falls at the same time as the sinus P wave). At the end of the recording, sinus rhythm accelerates, taking over cardiac rhythm again. A fusion beat (X) representing simultaneous ventricular activation by the ventricular ectopic beat and the conducted sinus rhythm is seen at the end of the AIVR.

Conclusion

AIVR.

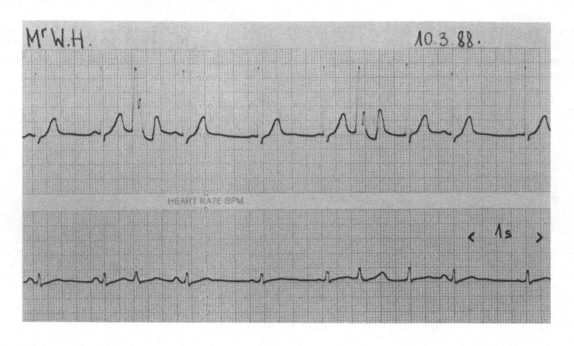

ECG no. 159: Mr. W.H., 42 years

Palpitations
No treatment
Holter ECG monitoring

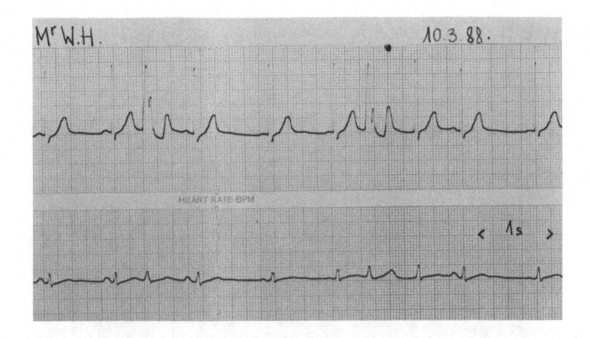

ECG no. 159: Mr. W.H., 42 years

Holter ECG monitoring

The first two complexes are of sinus origin. A wide QRS premature beat is interpolated between the second and third conducted sinus beats. A second interpolated VPB is seen after the fifth conducted sinus beat. That beat, by retrograde invasion in the AV conduction system, prolongs the PR interval of the next conducted sinus beat. The P wave is hidden in the T wave (•). The last complex is again a conducted sinus beat.

Conclusion

Interpolated extrasystole with concealed conduction.

133

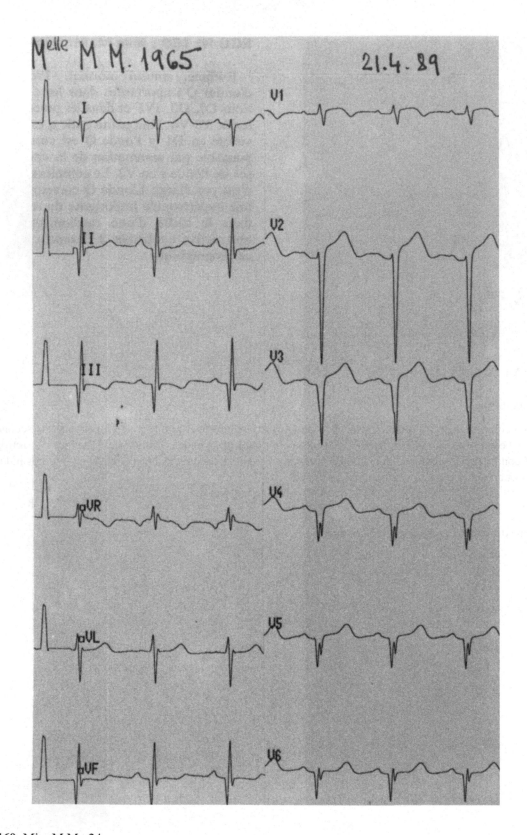

ECG no. 160: Miss M.M., 24 years

Hospitalized for pneumonia
No history of cardiac disease
(ECG donated by Dr. R.)

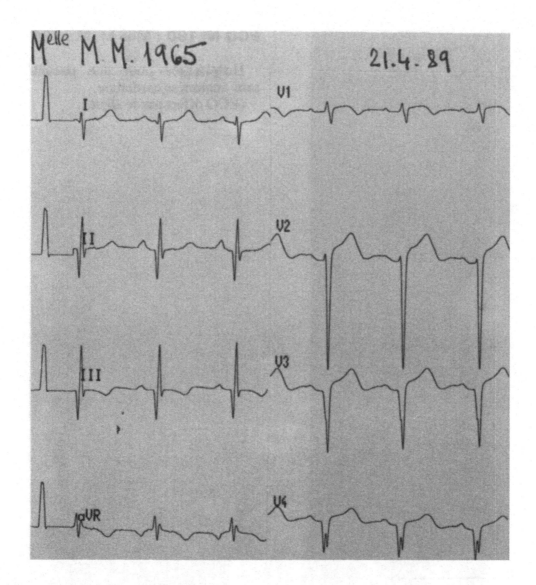

Melle M.M. 1965   21.4.89

ECG no. 160: Miss M.M., 24 years

Normal sinus rhythm. Deep Q waves are present in leads II, III, and aVF and in precordial leads V_3 to V_6. The QRS complex is not widened. These Q waves at this age suggest obstructive hypertrophic cardiomyopathy. The suspected etiology was confirmed by transthoracic ultrasound.

Conclusion

Hypertrophic cardiomyopathy.

135

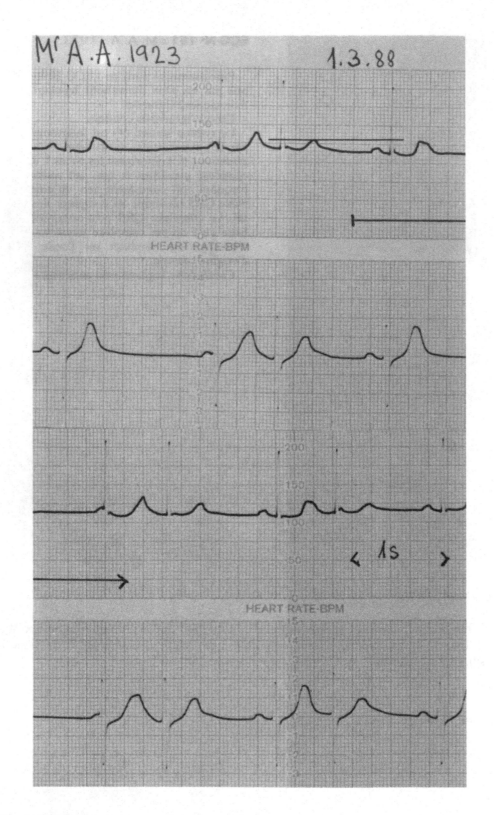

ECG no. 161: Mr. A.A., 65 years

Hypertension
Palpitations
Medication: diuretics
Continuous Holter ECG monitoring

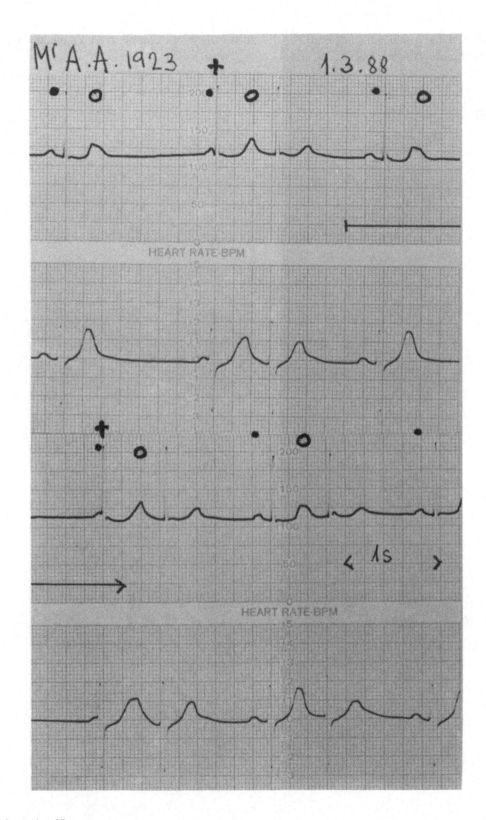

ECG no. 161: Mr. A.A., 65 years

Continuous Holter ECG monitoring

The sinus rhythm (•) is interrupted by atrial extrasystoles (bigeminy) (○). These atrial premature beats provoke a notching in the T waves of the previous QRS complex, and they are either blocked or conducted to the ventricle, with a QRS morphology identical to the conducted sinus beat. The first post-extrasystolic complex (X) is a junctional escape; it appears at the same time as the sinus P wave.

Conclusion

Atrial bigeminy.

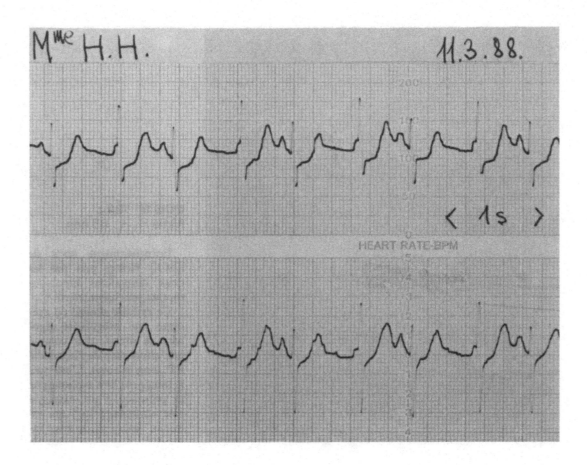

ECG no. 162: Mrs. H.H., 85 years

Palpitations
Heart failure
No digitalis
Holter ECG monitoring

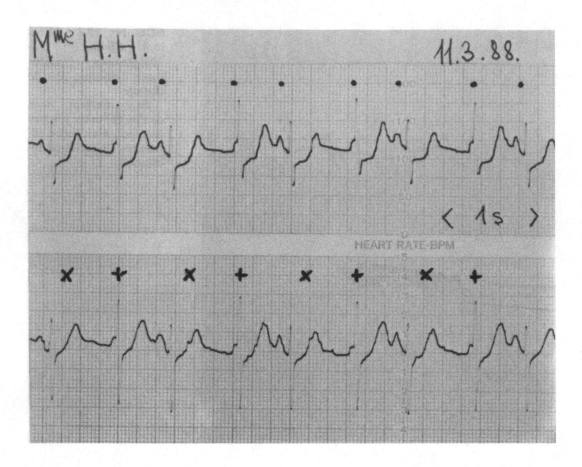

ECG no. 162: Mrs. H.H., 85 years

Holter ECG monitoring

The rhythm shows a regular irregularity, with a long–short R–R interval. Two explanations have to be considered.

1. An alternating PP interval (indicated by the dots) may be explained by the presence of sinus rhythm with a coupled atrial premature beat (X), which is seen more clearly in the inferior channel. This extrasystole is followed by a pause. The ventricular complex is the result of AV conduction with a prolonged PR, or the atrial extrasystole is blocked and followed by a junctional escape complex.
2. A sinus tachycardia is present with 3:2 Wenckebach conduction and marked AV prolongation of the second P wave.

Conclusion

No definite diagnosis is possible.

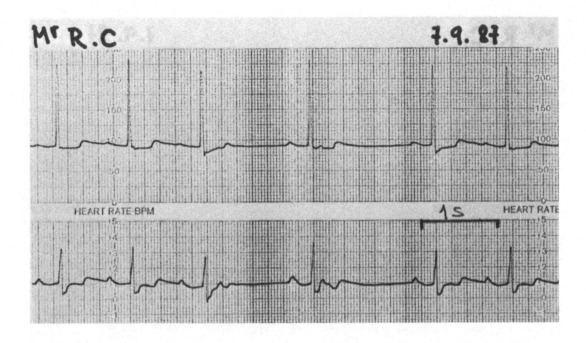

ECG no. 163: Mr. R.C., 60 years

Hypertension treated by diuretics
Holter ECG monitoring

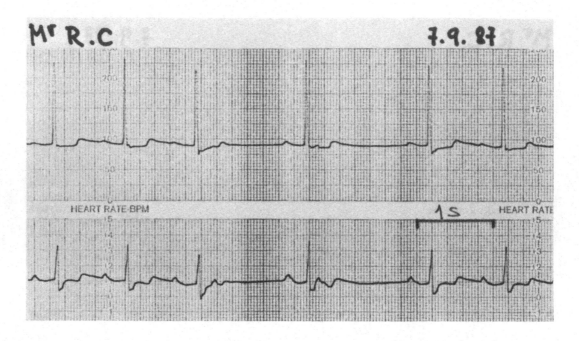

ECG no. 163: Mr. R.C., 60 years

Holter ECG monitoring

The first three complexes are conducted sinus beats with a prolonged PR interval of 0.32 s. Then, there is a blocked atrial premature beat modifying the ST segment and provoking a pause. The fourth complex is a conducted sinus beat, again with a blocked atrial premature beat in the ST segment. The last two complexes are conducted sinus beats; the first of which, after the pause, shows less PR prolongation than the second one.

Conclusion

Blocked atrial premature beats during sinus rhythm.

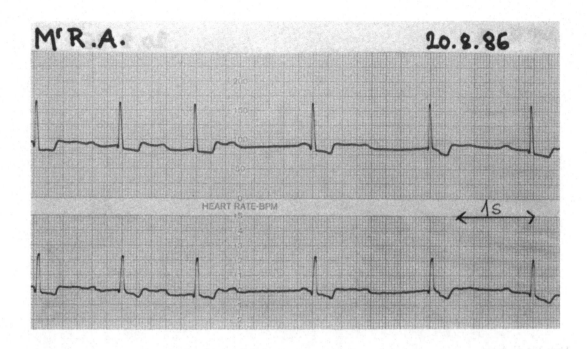

ECG no. 164: Mr. R.A.

Malaise
No known heart disease
Holter ECG monitoring

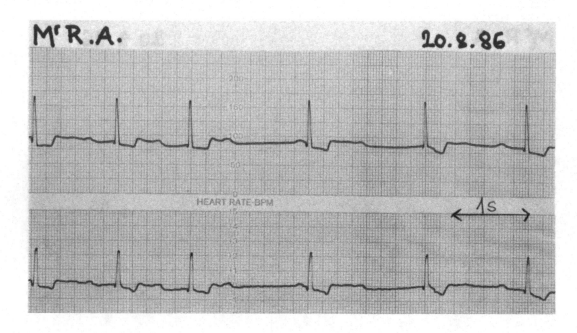

ECG no. 164: Mr. R.A.

Holter ECG monitoring

At the start of the recording, the prolonged PR interval shows a Wenckebach type of AV conduction. Following the P wave that is not conducted, we see a junctional escape (the P wave preceding this fourth complex is too close to the QRS to be conducted to the ventricle). Also, the next ventricular complex is of AV junctional origin. The last complex is a conducted sinus beat with a prolonged PR interval. The PP interval is modified by ventriculophasic behavior extending the PP interval when no P wave is present between ventricular complexes.

Conclusion

Type 1 second-degree AV block with Wenckebach phenomenon; junctional escapes; ventriculophasic P–P interval behavior.

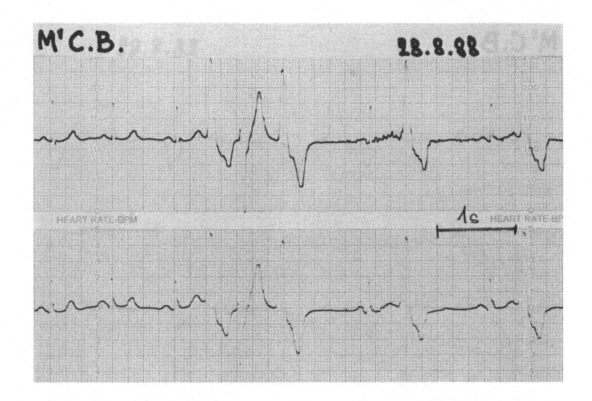

ECG no. 165: Mr. C.B., 56 years

History of myocardial infarction
Arterial hypertension
Palpitations
Treatment with aspirin
Holter ECG monitoring

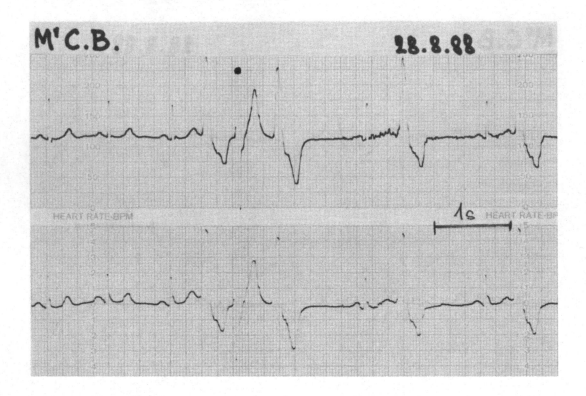

ECG no. 165: Mr. C.B., 56 years

Holter ECG monitoring

The first three conducted sinus beats are followed by three wide QRS complexes. At first glance, it looks like a run of ventricular tachycardia. Nevertheless, the middle complex (•) differs from the first and third complexes in QRS morphology. The middle one is preceded by a P wave, and its timing suggests a sinus origin. Therefore, it appears we are dealing with a conducted QRS with aberrant intraventricular conduction. Ventricular bigeminy is present following the last two conducted sinus beats.

Conclusion

Aberrant ventricular aberration giving the false appearance of a ventricular triplet.

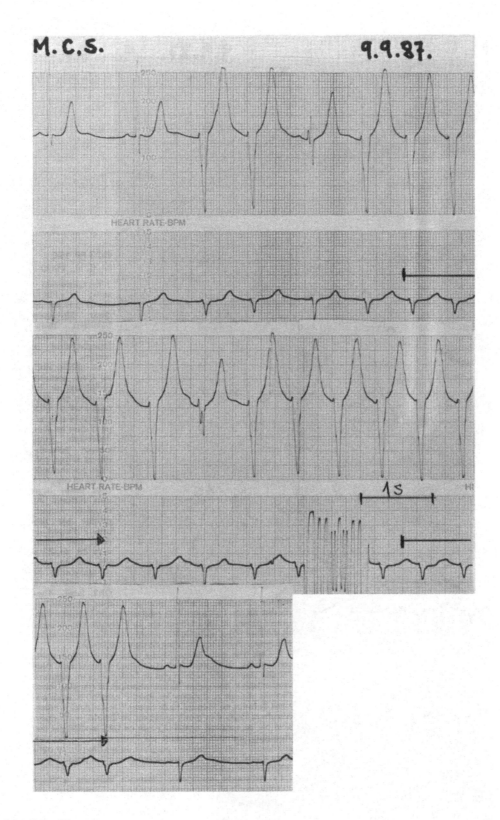

ECG no. 166: Mr. C.S., 87 years

Coronary artery disease
Palpitations with malaise
No treatment
Continuous Holter ECG monitoring

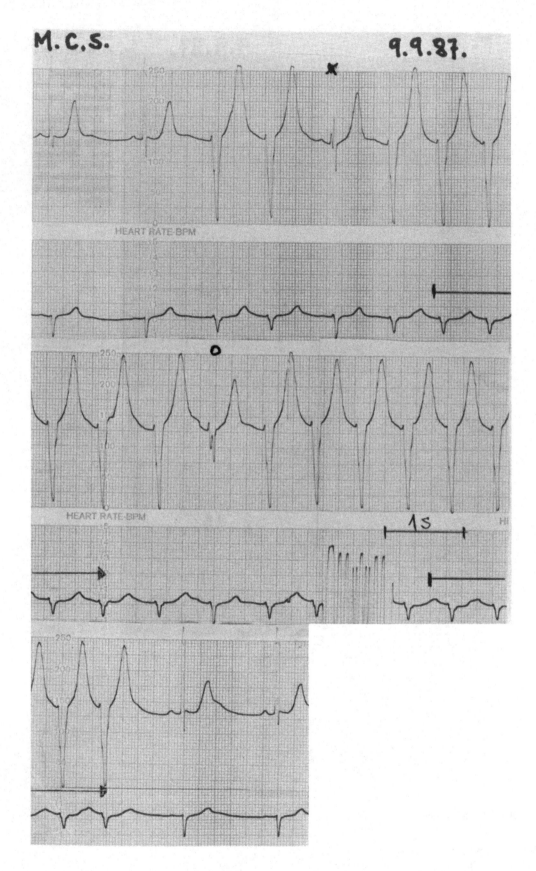

ECG no. 166: Mr. C.S., 87 years

Continuous Holter ECG monitoring

The first two conducted sinus beats are followed by two wide QRS complexes (0.14 s); these two complexes appear prematurely and are not preceded by a P wave. Then, we see a QRS complex different from the conducted sinus beat but narrower than the third and fourth complexes. This beat is preceded by a sinus P wave and has the same PR interval as the first two conducted sinus beats (X). It is a fusion complex with minimal contribution to ventricular excitation from the ectopic ventricular rhythm. We then see a run of tachycardia of 15 wide QRS complexes. The seventh complex of this tachycardia is different in morphology (○) and preceded by a P wave, representing another fusion beat. At the end, the ventricular tachycardia stops and a conducted sinus rhythm reappears.

Conclusion

A relatively slow nonsustained monomorphic ventricular tachycardia with fusion beats because of intermittent AV conduction following a sinus P wave.

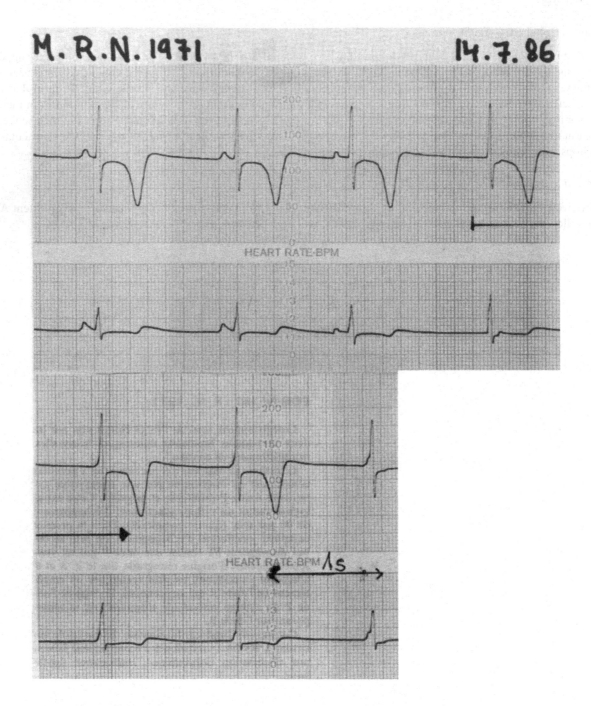

ECG no. 167: Mr. R.N., 15 years

Patient known for status post mitral valve replacement and status post tricuspid valvuloplasty
Digitalis
Continuous Holter ECG monitoring

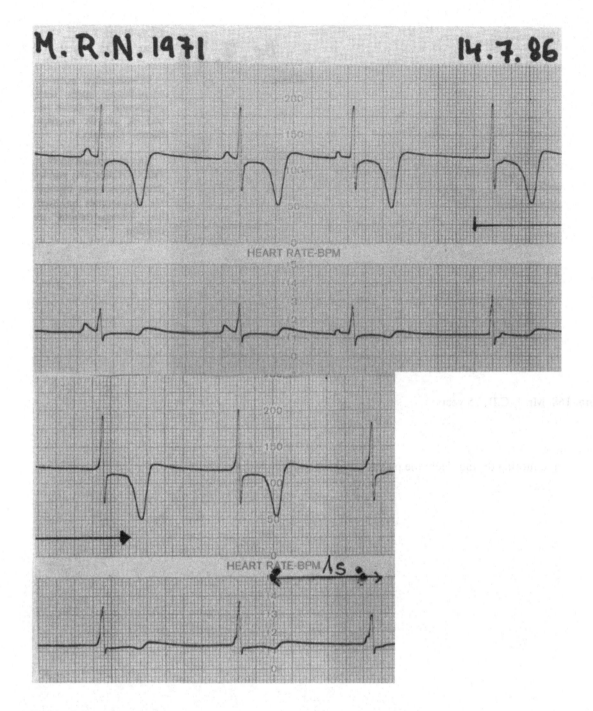

ECG no. 167: Mr. R.N., 15 years

Continuous Holter ECG monitoring

The slow sinus rhythm (39 bpm) seen in the first two complexes is interrupted by an atrial premature beat (the P wave of the third complex is different from those before the first and second QRS). This premature beat induces an escape junctional rhythm of 40 bpm (four complexes). In the second, third, and fourth junctional complexes, there is a change in the initial part of the R wave. This is caused by the P wave of the sinus rhythm, which reappears and superimposes itself on the R wave.

Conclusion

Sinus bradycardia; atrial extrasystole; junctional escape rhythm; possible digitalis intoxication.

151

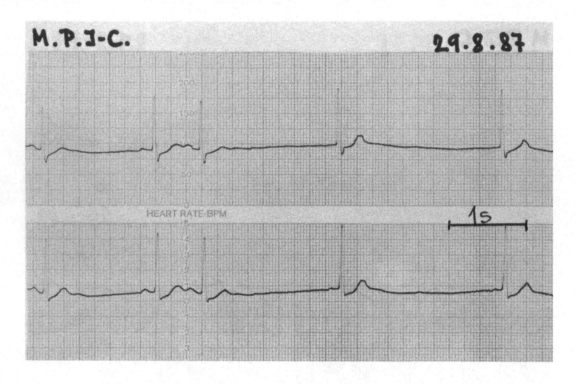

ECG no. 168: Mr. J.-C.P., 75 years

Malaise
No medication
Holter ECG monitoring during sleep; the patient therefore is asymptomatic

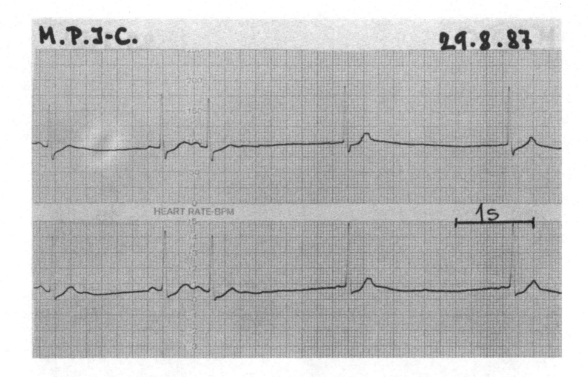

ECG no. 168: Mr. J.-C.P., 75 years

Holter ECG monitoring

The first two complexes show sinus bradycardia at 40 bpm. The atrial extrasystole that follows worsens the bradycardia. The fourth and fifth QRS complexes represent AV junctional escape beats at 30 bpm.

Conclusion

Sinus node dysfunction.

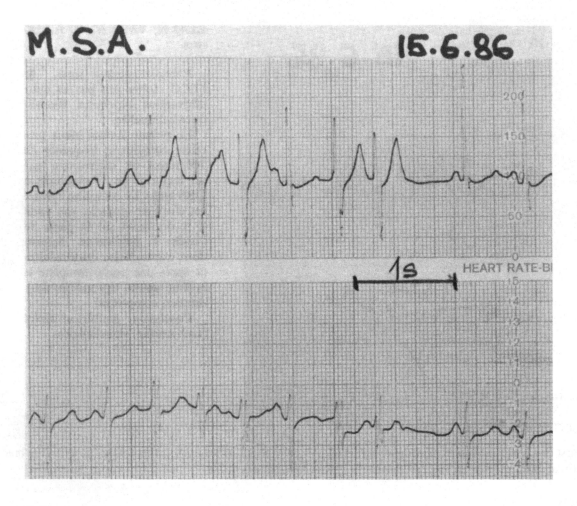

ECG no. 169: Mr. S.A., 56 years

Coronary artery disease
Holter ECG monitoring

154

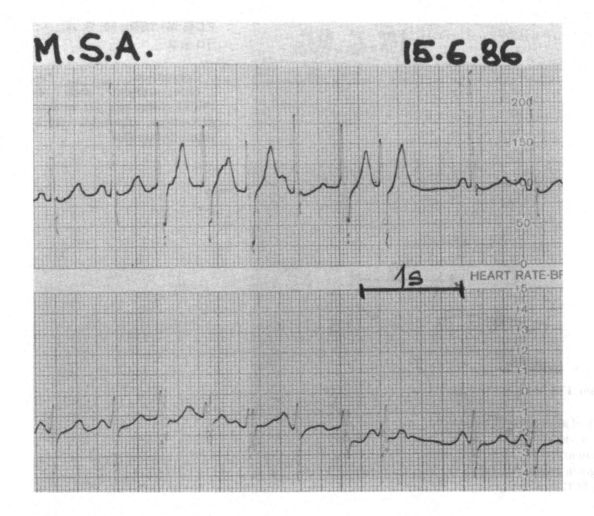

ECG no. 169: Mr. S.A., 56 years

Holter ECG monitoring

Following two conducted sinus P waves with an interval of 600 ms (sinus tachycardia), there are three wide QRS complexes with AV dissociation. The next complex is of sinus origin, as the P wave is seen in the descent of the T wave of the previous QRS. We then have two ventricular extrasystoles followed by conducted sinus rhythm.

Conclusion

Ventricular triplet and doublet.

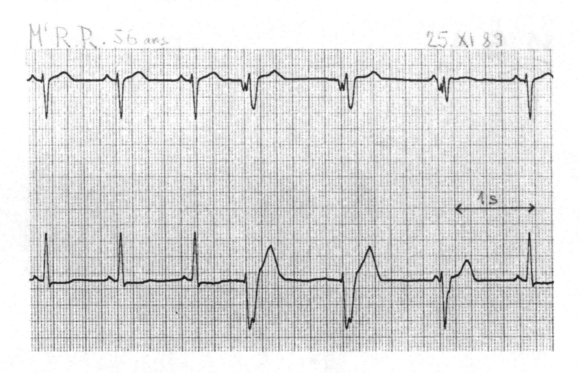

ECG no. 170: Mr. R.R., 56 years

History of myocardial infarction
Anterior aneurysm
Palpitations
No digoxin treatment
Holter ECG monitoring

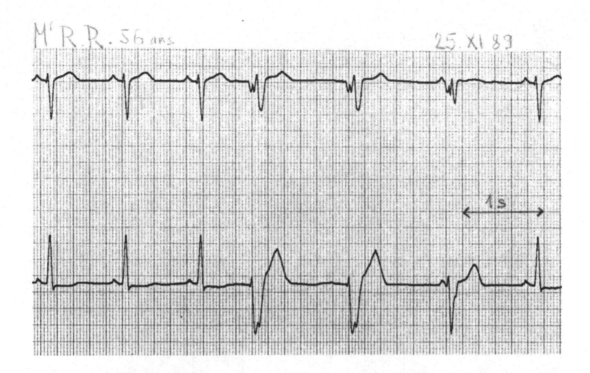

ECG no. 170: Mr. R.R., 56 years

Holter ECG monitoring

The first three complexes are of sinus origin. We then see two wide QRS complexes (0.20 s). The fifth QRS is similar in morphology, but its duration decreases to 0.14 s and it has a sinus P wave in front. However, the PR interval is much shorter than that of the conducted sinus beats. The last complex is again a conducted sinus beat. The beats with a wide QRS represent an AIVR. The third complex of this rhythm shows fusion between the AIVR and the sinus rhythm. The sinus activity is not interrupted but slows down slightly. The P waves occur in the QRS–T complex of the first two beats of the AIVR; therefore, they fall in the refractory period of the ventricle and cannot be conducted.

Conclusion

AIVR.

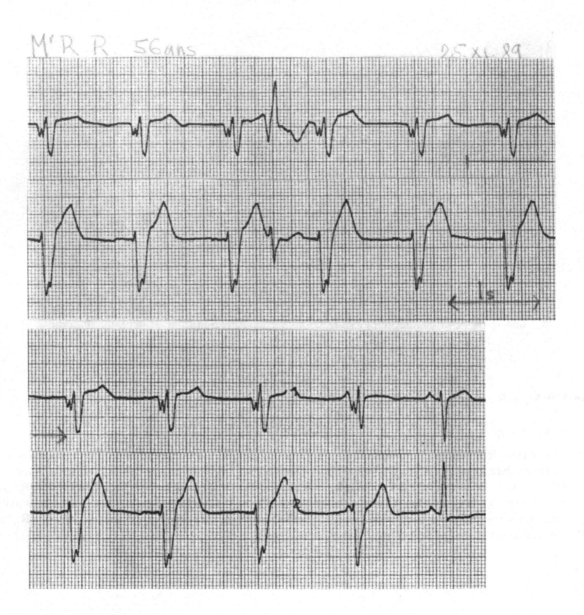

ECG no. 171: Mr. R.R., 56 years

History of myocardial infarction
Anterior aneurysm
Palpitations
No digoxin treatment
Holter ECG continuous monitoring

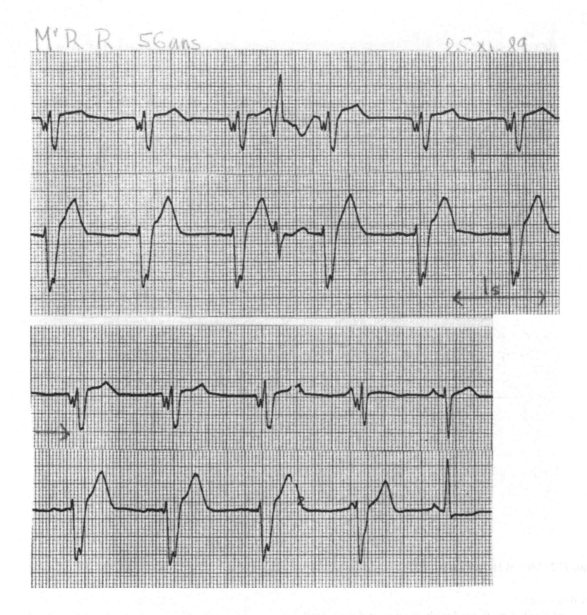

ECG no. 171: Mr. R.R., 56 years

Holter ECG continuous monitoring

The tracing predominantly shows wide QRS complexes ending with a sinus P wave conducted to the ventricle. The wide QRS complexes represent an AIVR. The changes in T wave height suggest the presence of (nonconducted) sinus P waves during AIVR. The fourth QRS has a different configuration and is most likely a captured sinus beat with right bundle branch block. The last QRS of the AIVR has a sinus P wave in front. The QRS configuration is slightly different from the previous one, suggesting some fusion with a conducted sinus P wave.

Conclusion

AIVR.

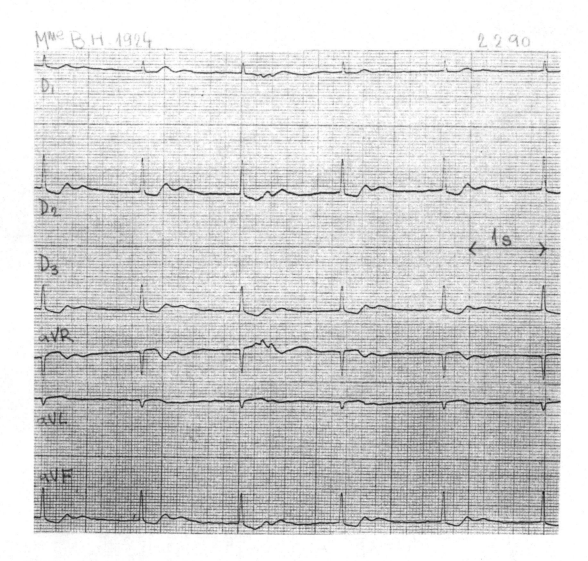

ECG no. 172: Mrs. B.H., 66 years

Mitral valve disease
Known atrial fibrillation treated with digoxin and verapamil

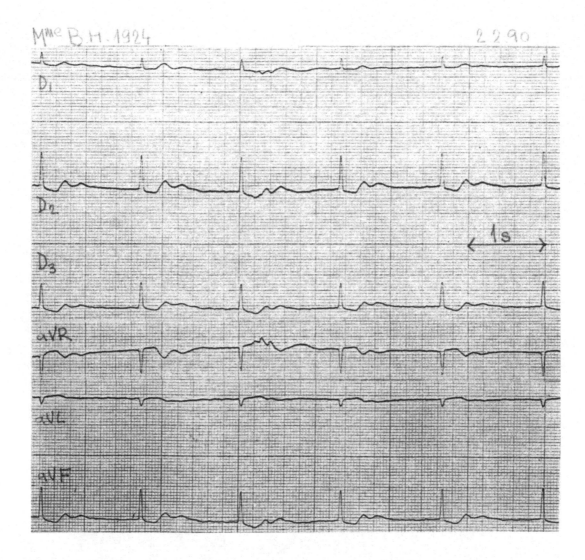

D₁

D₂

1 s

D₃

aVR

aVL

aVF

ECG no. 172: Mrs. B.H., 66 years

The tracing shows regular, narrow QRS complexes without P waves preceding them. The atrial activity is not seen clearly, but the baseline is undulating and these waves seem to be fast. These features suggest underlying atrial fibrillation with complete AV block and a junctional escape rhythm with a rate of 45 bpm.

Conclusion

Atrial fibrillation with complete AV block and a junctional escape rhythm. The effect of the digoxin, potentiated by the presence of verapamil, is probably the reason for this AV block.

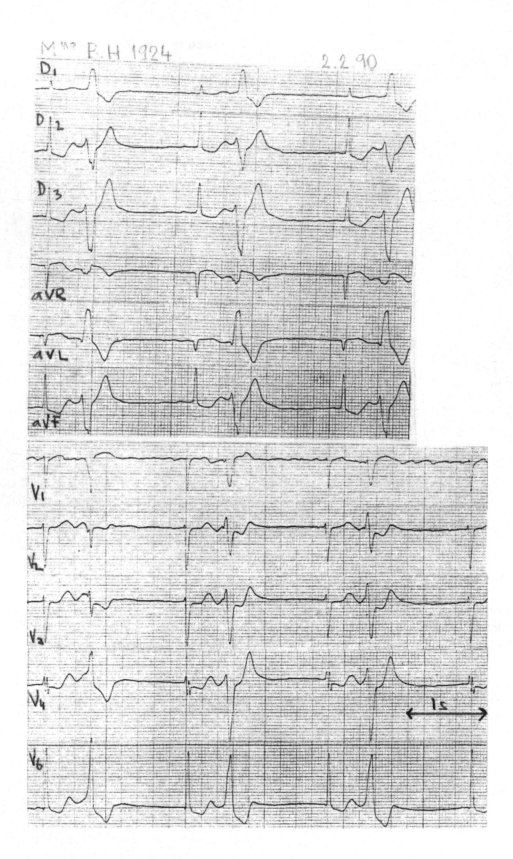

ECG no. 173: Mrs. B.H., 66 years

Mitral valve disease
Known atrial fibrillation treated with digoxin and verapamil

162

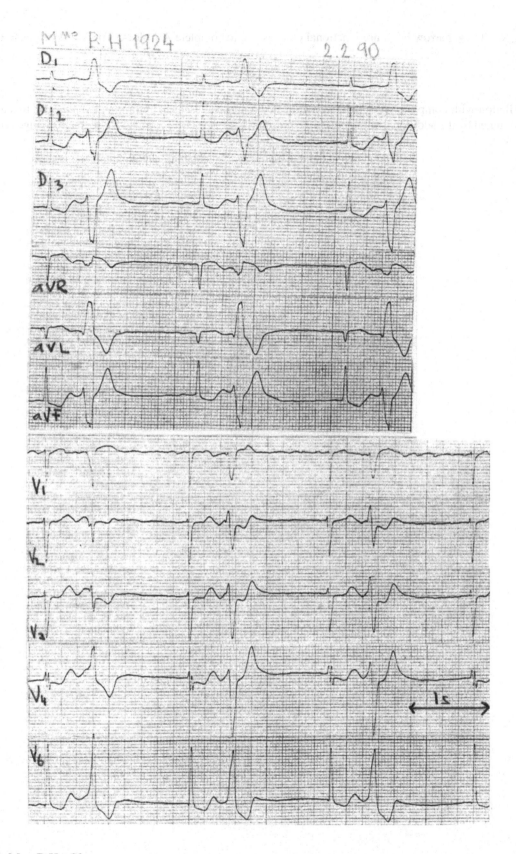

ECG no. 173: Mrs. B.H., 66 years

Atrial fibrillation is present at the atrial level. At the ventricular level, a narrow QRS is followed by a wide one, with a left bundle branch block-like configuration. These coupled VPBs are followed by a pause of a fixed length, which is terminated

163

by a narrow QRS. These narrow beats are junctional escapes due to complete AV block. The VPBs originate from the right ventricle.

Conclusion

Atrial fibrillation with complete AV block, a complicated junctional escape rhythm, and ventricular bigeminy. Digoxin treatment potentiated by the additional verapamil is the most likely cause. There are also ST segment changes consistent with digoxin treatment.

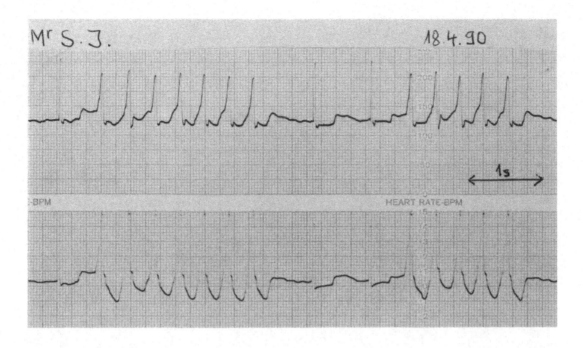

ECG no. 174: Mr. S.J., 61 years

Palpitations
Malaise
Holter ECG monitoring

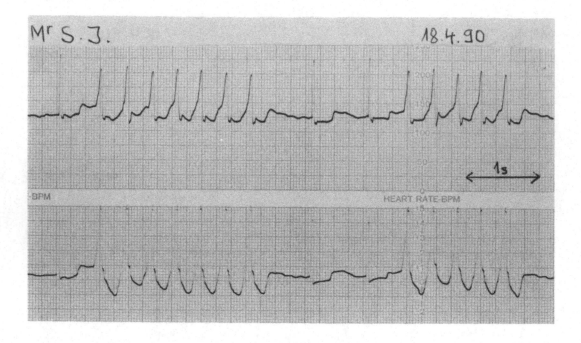

ECG no. 174: Mr. S.J., 61 years

Holter ECG monitoring

The atrial rhythm is atrial fibrillation. At the ventricular level, a narrow QRS is followed by a seven-beat nonsustained ventricular tachycardia; then, we again see two narrow QRS and a new onset of ventricular tachycardia of five QRS. The tachycardia appears monomorphic, with a heart rate of 170 bpm.

Conclusion

Atrial fibrillation; nonsustained ventricular tachycardia with runs of seven and five QRS.

NB: For tachycardia to be defined as sustained, it must last longer than 30 s (arbitrary limit), or less than 30 s if the patient collapses because of hemodynamic failure.

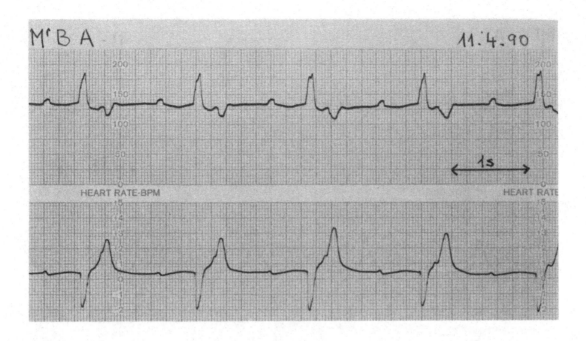

ECG no. 175: Mr. B.A., 64 years

Shortness of breath during exercise
No medication
Holter ECG monitoring

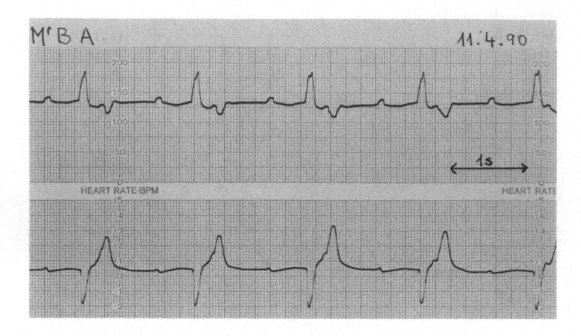

ECG no. 175: Mr. B.A., 64 years

Holter ECG monitoring

The atrial activity is of sinus origin and regular, with a rate of 75 bpm. Every second P wave is hidden in the ST segment of the QRS complex. The ventricular complexes are wide and have a morphology of bundle branch block and a rate of 35 bpm. There is no relation between the P wave and the QRS complex, indicating complete AV block.

Conclusion

Complete AV block.

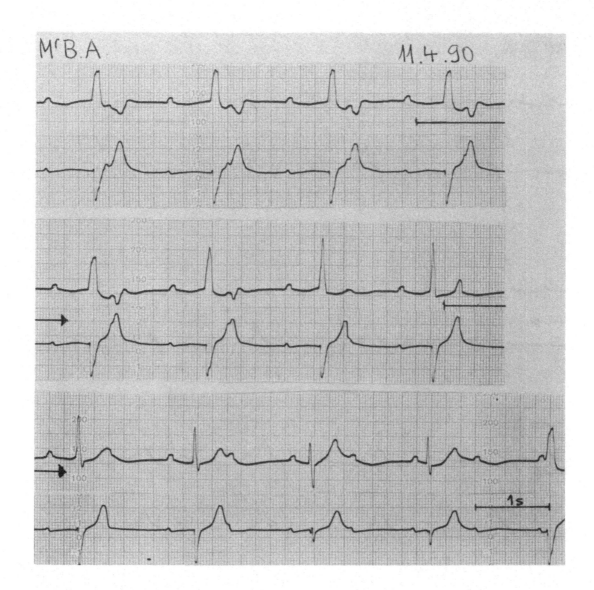

ECG no. 176: Mr. B.A., 64 years

Shortness of breath during exercise
No medication
Holter ECG continuous monitoring

169

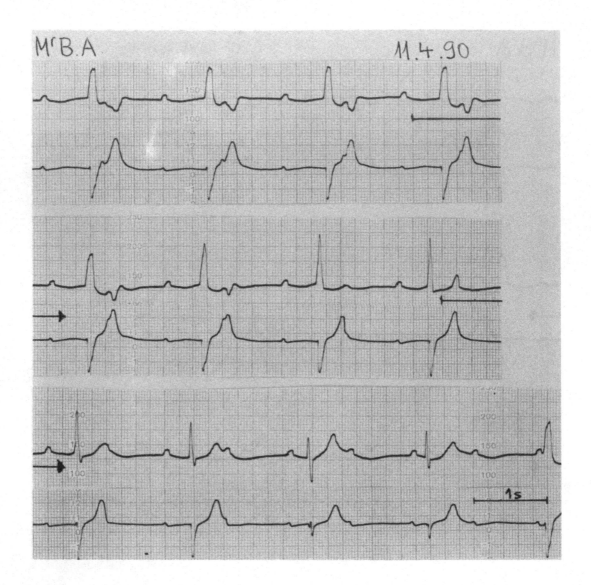

ECG no. 176: Mr. B.A., 64 years

Holter ECG continuous monitoring

Atrial activity is seen, with regular P waves of sinus origin at a rate of 74 bpm. A ventriculophasic phenomenon slightly extends the PP distance between the two atrial waves when no ventricular complex is in between. The ventricular complexes at the beginning of the recording have a wide QRS morphology with a bundle branch block appearance and a heart rate of 38 bpm. The sixth, seventh, and eighth complexes become narrower; an S wave appears in the ninth QRS complex that becomes deeper in the QRS complexes thereafter and changes its morphology, and we see an S wave that becomes progressively deeper and deeper in the first channel. The last QRS complex of the recording also has a wide QRS with the same type of morphology as seen at the beginning of the recording. The ventricular heart rate varies very little; it accelerates slightly between the sixth and eighth complexes, and then slows again to become the same as at the beginning of the tracing. The P waves do not conduct to the ventricles. The ventricular rhythm is an escape rhythm with a left bundle branch morphology in the first five ventricular beats. The gradual narrowing of the escape rhythm thereafter is difficult to explain without a His bundle electrogram. It may be the result of fusion between escape rhythms in both bundle branches.

Conclusion

Complete AV block. We suggest the possibility of two escape rhythms that interact with each other, resulting in fusion of the escape beat.

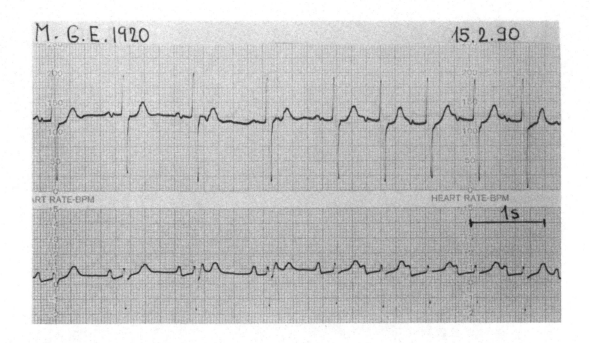

ECG no. 177: Mr. G.E., 70 years

Aortic valve disease
Mitral valve disease
No medication
No signs of cardiac insufficiency
Holter ECG monitoring

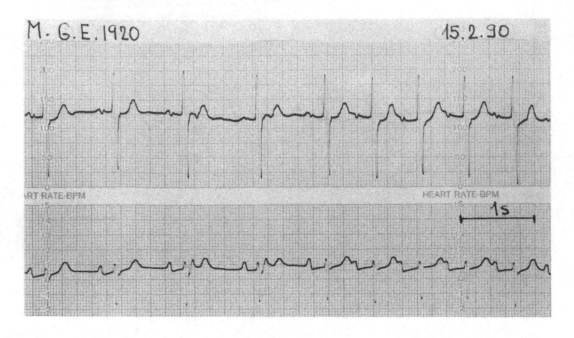

ECG no. 177: Mr. G.E., 70 years

Holter ECG monitoring

The first five complexes are of sinus origin and accelerate slowly over time. Analyzing the ST segment of the third and fourth complexes, one may recognize an ectopic P wave not conducted to the ventricle. After the fifth complex, we see another ectopic P wave, which is more delayed in its appearance and this time conducts to the ventricles and initiates an atrial tachycardia with a heart rate of around 100 bpm. The PR interval during tachycardia is slightly extended.

Conclusion

Atrial extrasystoles, blocked at first, then followed by the onset of an atrial tachycardia.

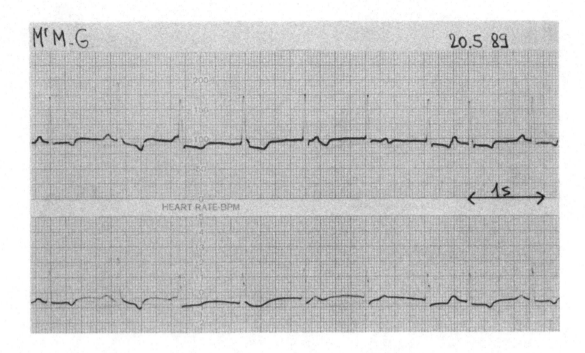

ECG no. 178: Mr. M.G., 52 years

Angina pectoris
Palpitations
Holter ECG monitoring

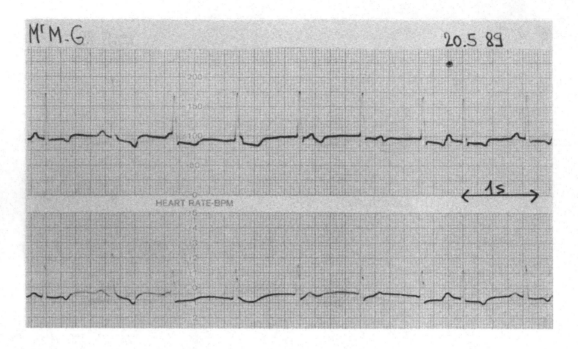

ECG no. 178: Mr. M.G., 52 years

Holter ECG monitoring

The conducted sinus rhythm of the first two complexes is followed by a QRS complex similar to the two previous ones seen during conducted sinus rhythm. The following four QRS complexes are identical, their heart rate is 70 bpm, and they are not preceded by a P wave. The P waves of sinus origin, which have a slightly slower heart rate, appear in the QRS complexes, especially in the ST segments and T waves. They remain blocked because of the refractory period in the AV conduction. The next sinus P wave (•) occurs later and can therefore be conducted to the ventricle, interrupting the accelerated junctional rhythm. The PR interval of the conducted beat is prolonged because of retrograde invasion of the junctional beat. The last complex also is of sinus origin.

Conclusion

Accelerated AV junctional rhythm.

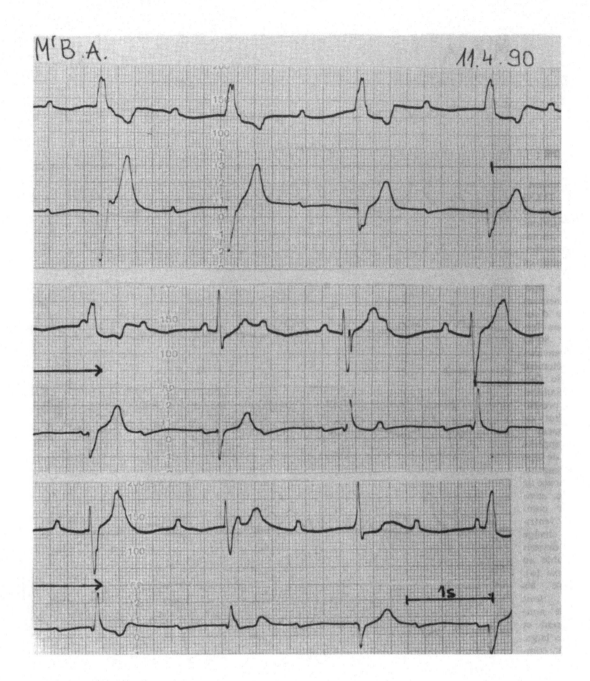

ECG no. 179: Mr. B.A., 64 years

Shortness of breath
No medication
Continuous Holter ECG monitoring

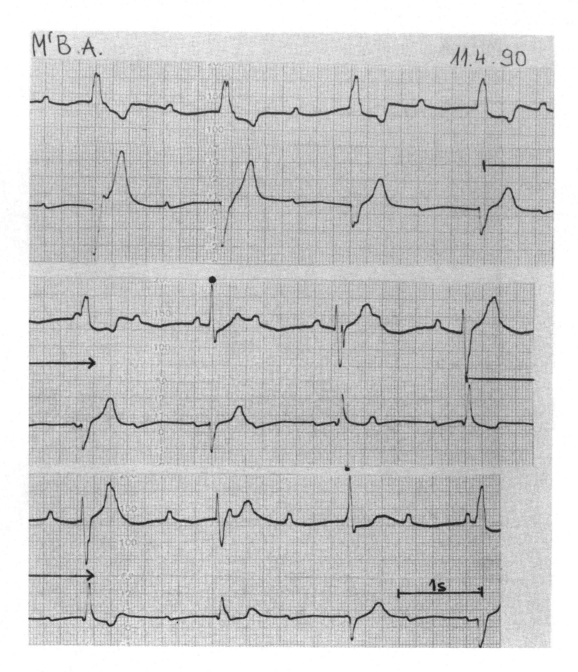

ECG no. 179: Mr. B.A., 64 years

Continuous Holter ECG monitoring

There is sinus rhythm with a heart rate of 80 to 85 bpm. The P waves are completely dissociated from the ventricular complexes. The QRS at the beginning of the tracing is wide and has a left bundle branch block morphology. Without a change in rate, the QRS configuration gradually changes, becoming less wide with the sixth ventricular complex (•) and showing further narrowing and a configuration similar to the 11th complex (•). Between these two complexes, the QRS configuration, axis, and width are different. The last QRS is quite similar to the first, especially to the third complex in the tracing. These modifications in the appearance of the ventricular complexes may be explained best by the presence of two escape rhythms in the bundle branches with approximately the same rate and different degrees of fusion.

Conclusion

Complete AV block with two escape rhythms with a nearly similar heart rate, inducing fusion.

176

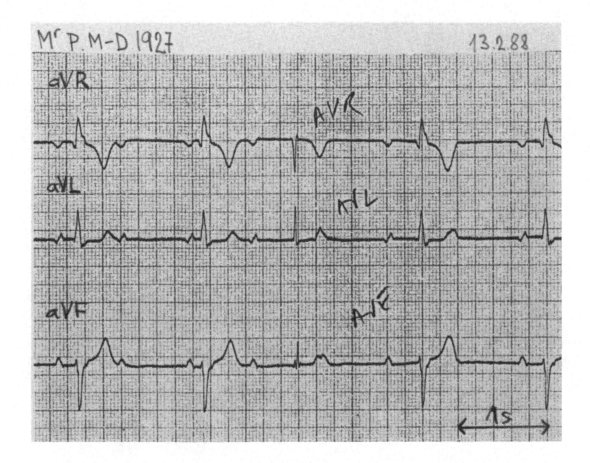

ECG no. 180: Mr. P.-M.D., 61 years

Syncope with loss of consciousness
No medical treatment

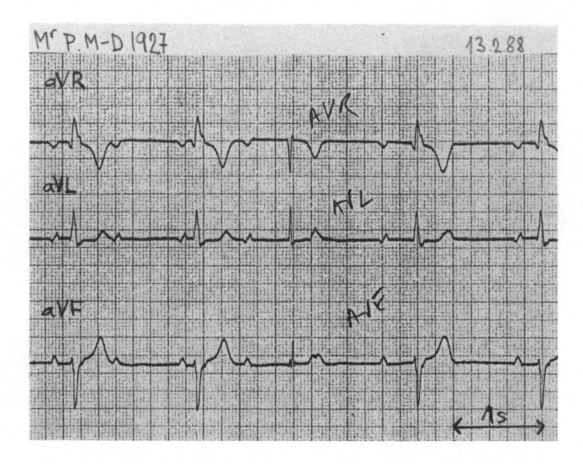

ECG no. 180: Mr. P.-M.D., 61 years

The P waves are of sinus origin; their rate is 82 bpm. The ventricular complexes are wide, are independent of the atrial rhythm, and have a slow regular activity, with a rate of 45 bpm, with the exception of the third QRS complex, which is narrow and comes earlier. That beat is a conducted QRS with a prolonged PR interval. Of interest is the discrete irregularity of the P waves, which may be explained by the ventriculophasic phenomenon (the interval between two P waves being longer when there is no ventricular complex in between).

Conclusion

Advanced AV block with one sinus capture and ventriculophasic alternans of the PP interval.

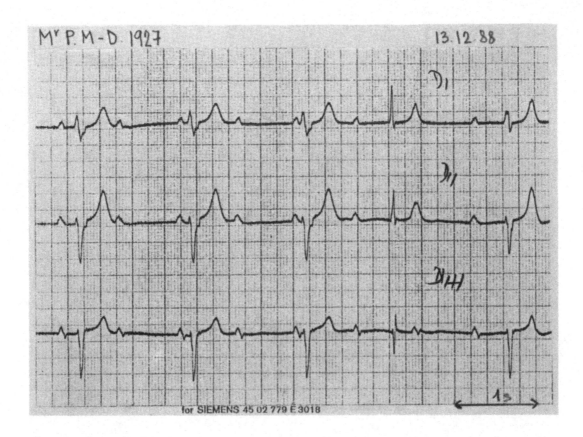

ECG no. 181: Mr. P.-M.D., 61 years

Shortness of breath on exercise
Loss of consciousness
No medical treatment

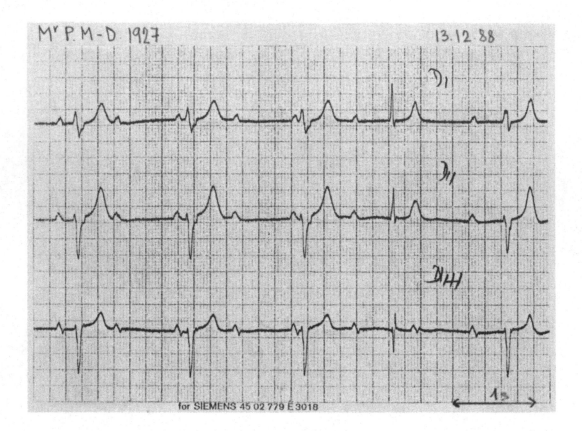

ECG no. 181: Mr. P.-M.D., 61 years

Regular atrial activity of sinus origin, with a rate of 80 bpm. The ventricular rhythm shows wide QRS complexes (0.14 s), regular, with a rate of 42 bpm. There is no relation between the atrial and ventricular rhythms, except in the fourth ventricular complex, which is narrow and the result of AV conduction with a markedly prolonged PR interval.

Conclusion

Advanced AV block with one conducted sinus beat.

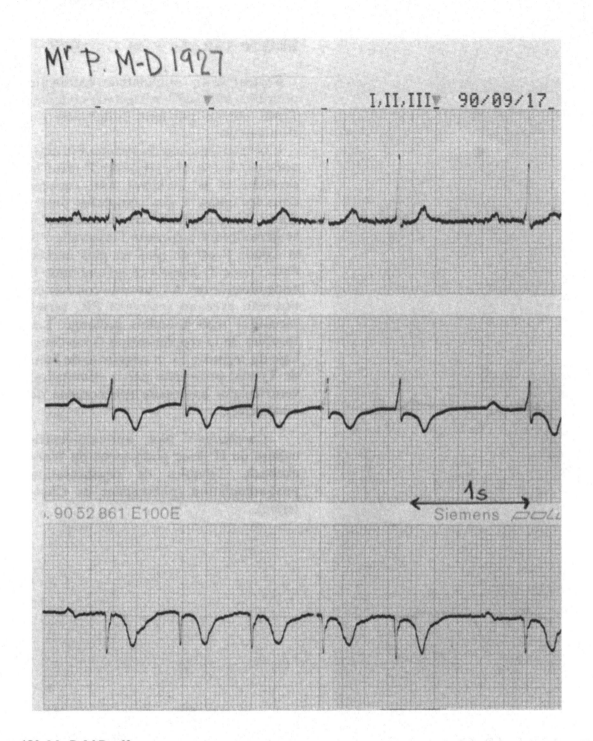

ECG no. 182: Mr. P.-M.D., 63 years

Patient with permanent endocavitary stimulation (pacemaker)
Pacemaker implanted for complete AV block, as diagnosed on ECG nos. 180 and 181
Recording obtained during inhibition of the pacemaker

181

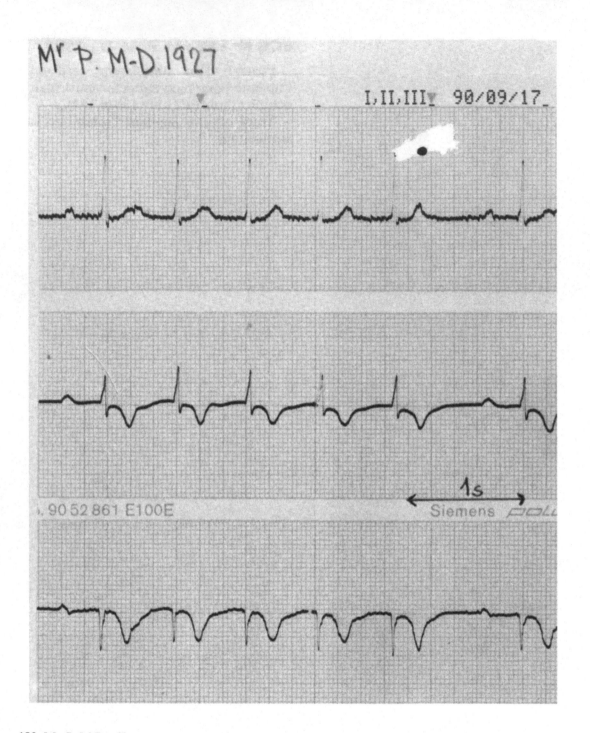

ECG no. 182: Mr. P.-M.D., 63 years

Patient with permanent endocavitary stimulation (pacemaker) for complete AV block

Recording obtained during inhibition of the pacemaker

Sinus tachycardia is present, with Wenckebach conduction to the ventricle. The P waves, except for the first and last one, are hidden in the T waves. Finally, a P wave is blocked (•). The next P wave conducts again with a PR interval shortened in comparison with the PR interval of the last previously conducted beat. There are deep negative T waves in leads II and III; these are called the "memory sign" following pacing in the right ventricular apex (Chatterjee phenomenon).

Conclusion

Second-degree AV block with Wenckebach phenomenon, repolarization alterations post endocavitary permanent stimulation (Chatterjee phenomenon).

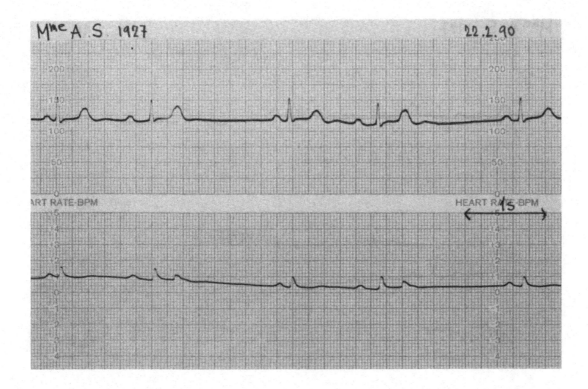

ECG no. 183: Mrs. A.S., 63 years

Malaise
Palpitations
Holter ECG monitoring

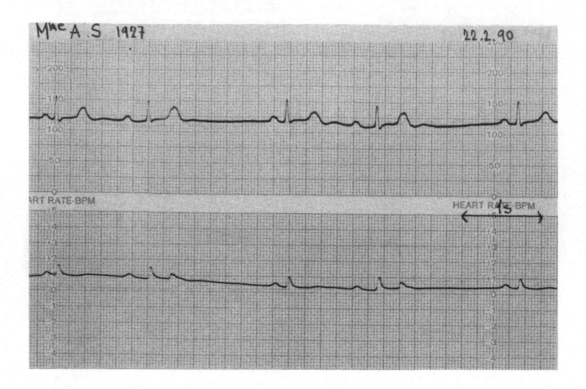

ECG no. 183: Mrs. A.S., 63 years

Holter ECG monitoring

Sinus bradycardia (58 bpm) interrupted after two complexes by a pause that is less than twice the previous RR interval. The reason for the pause is AV block of the atrial deflection located in the T wave of the second complex. The PR interval of the complexes, which are conducted to the ventricles, increases: the first one is 0.16 s and the last one 0.28 s. This suggests either second-degree AV block with Wenckebach conduction interrupted by the blocked premature atrial beat or termination of the pause by an AV junctional escape. In the latter situation, the P wave before the escape is not conducted to the ventricle.

Conclusion

Sinus bradycardia with blocked atrial premature beats.

184

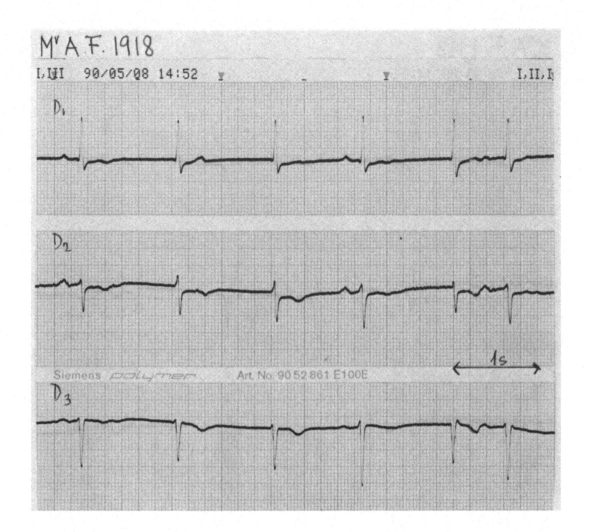

ECG no. 184: Mr. A.F., 72 years

Arterial hypertension
Malaise
Weakness
Medication: diltiazem

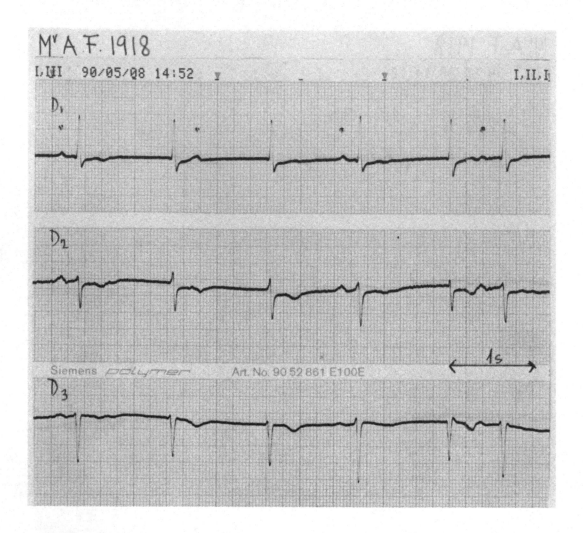

ECG no. 184: Mr. A.F., 72 years

Severe sinus bradycardia. The sinus P waves, which can be identified in the tracing (•), have a rate of 35 bpm. These P waves conduct to the ventricle in the first, fourth, and sixth complexes. The second, third, and fifth ventricular complexes are the result of a junctional escape rhythm with an interval of 1,200 ms.

Conclusion

Sick sinus syndrome with junctional escapes. The medication may have played an important role in slowing down the sinus rhythm.

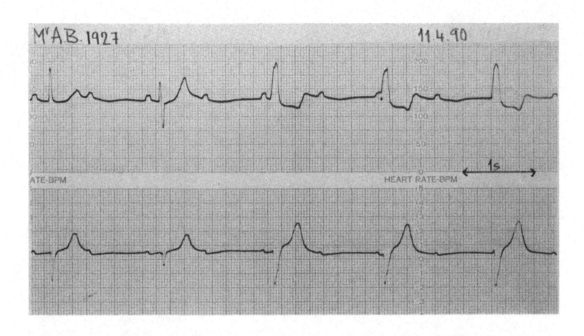

ECG no. 185: Mr. A.B., 63 years

Syncope
No treatment
Holter ECG monitoring

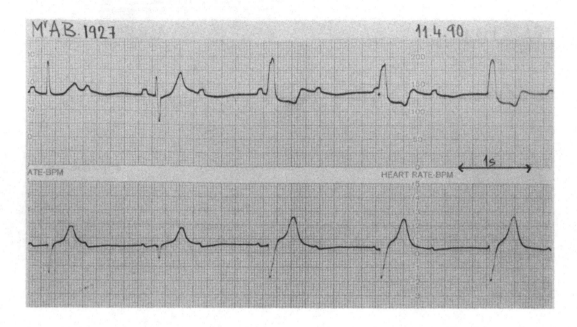

ECG no. 185: Mr. A.B., 63 years

Holter ECG monitoring

On this tracing, there are sinus P waves with a rate of 72 bpm. There is no relation between atrial and ventricular events. The ventricular rhythm has identical R–R intervals with a rate of 38 bpm but different QRS morphologies. The first ventricular complex has a QRS configuration between it and the QRS in beats two and three. In view of this behavior without a change in the R–R intervals during the tracing, we postulate escape competition between the two bundle branches at approximately the same escape rate, resulting in the possibility of fusion beats. At the atrial level, ventriculophasic P–P alternation is present: the interval between the two P waves, with no ventricular complexes between them, is slightly longer than the interval of the two P waves embracing a ventricular complex.

Conclusion

Complete AV block with fusion between two escape sites; ventriculophasic P–P interval alternans.

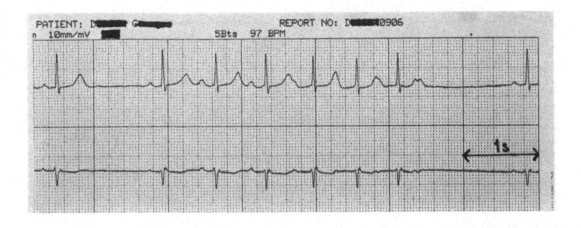

ECG no. 186: Mr. D.G., 82 years

Palpitations
Amiodarone
Holter ECG monitoring

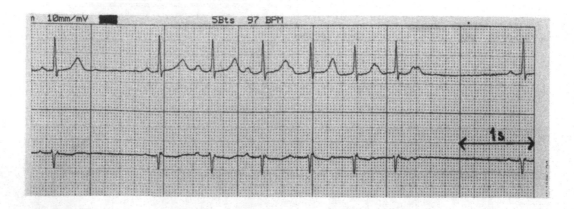

ECG no. 186: Mr. D.G., 82 years

Holter ECG monitoring

A sinus bradycardia is present in the first two complexes, with a rate of 42 bpm. This is followed by an episode of rapid atrial rhythm. The P waves during that episode are different from the sinus P waves, indicating an ectopic atrial tachycardia. The atrial rate of the tachycardia accelerates progressively, from 82 bpm at the beginning of the tachycardia to 100 bpm at the end. This is accompanied by an increasing delay in AV conduction (the PR interval goes from 0.20 s at the beginning of the arrhythmia to 0.28 s at the end), with the P wave increasingly more hidden in the preceding T wave. The last P wave is blocked, and the sinus bradycardia reappears.

Conclusion

Sinus bradycardia and a paroxysmal episode of atrial tachycardia.

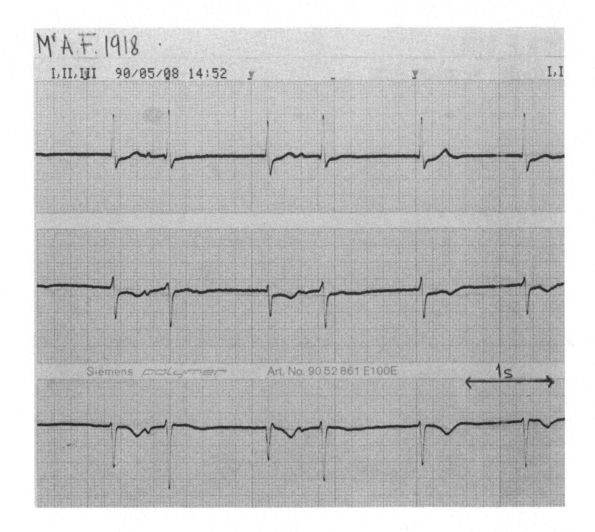

ECG no. 187: Mr. A.F., 72 years

Arterial hypertension
Malaise
Weakness
Diltiazem
Holter ECG monitoring

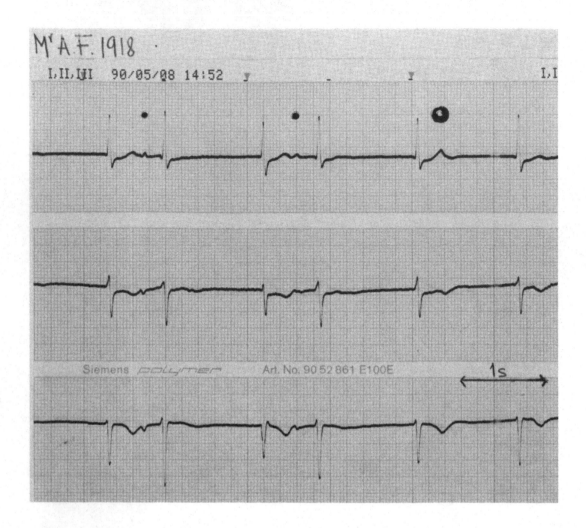

ECG no. 187: Mr. A.F., 72 years

Holter ECG monitoring

An irregular ventricular rhythm is present with a few P waves. The P wave configuration is negative in leads II and III, arguing against an origin in the sinus node. There clearly is an AV junctional rhythm with identical R–R intervals following the second, fourth, and fifth QRS. The question arises as to whether the P waves are caused by retrograde conduction to the atrium after junctional beats 1 and 3. These P waves are followed by conduction to the ventricle. Are they an example of a so-called escape capture bigeminy following the junctional rhythm? What argues against it is the third P wave, which is located on top of the T wave following QRS 5 (○). We therefore conclude that the P waves are not related to the junctional rhythm but arise independently low in the right atrium. The first two P waves are conducted to the ventricle with slight ventricular aberrancy.

Conclusion

Atrial bradycardia with an escape junctional rhythm. Diltiazem treatment may have contributed to the arrhythmia.

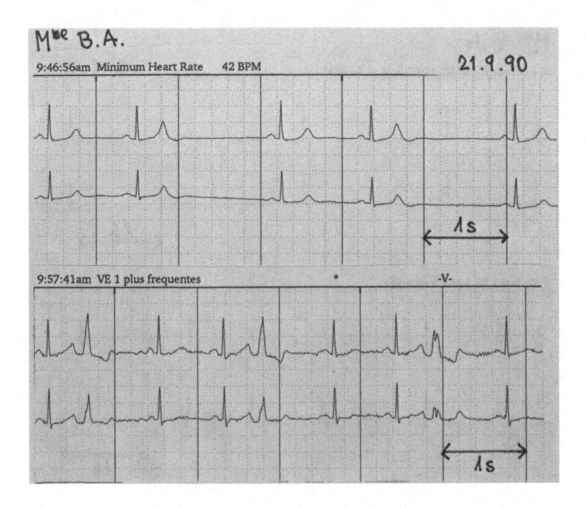

ECG no. 188: Mrs. B.A., 53 years

Palpitations
No treatment
Holter ECG monitoring

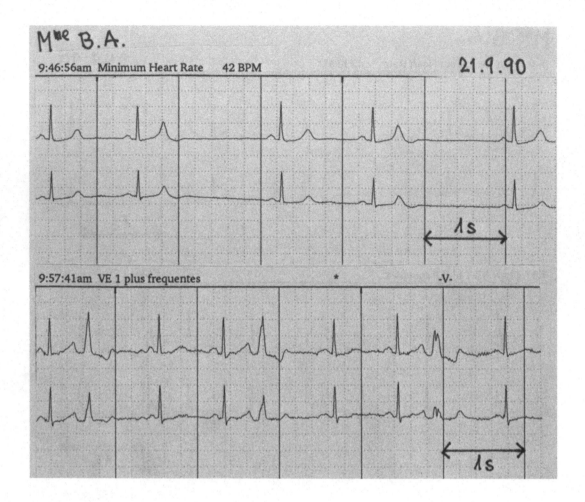

ECG no. 188: Mrs. B.A., 53 years

Holter ECG monitoring

    In the *upper tracing*, a conducted sinus rhythm of around 55 bpm is followed by two pauses. The T waves of the second and fourth ventricular complexes are taller because of a superimposed atrial premature beat, which is not conducted to the ventricle. Therefore, the pauses are a result of the blocked atrial premature beats. In the *lower tracing*, the sinus rhythm accelerates slightly to 78 bpm. After the first, third, and fifth sinus complexes, there is a premature wide QRS complex. The T wave of the previous complex hides a premature P wave. Note the difference from the previous T wave, which is not followed by the premature beat. The wide QRS complex therefore is the conducted atrial premature beat, and the width of the ventricular complex is the result of an intraventricular aberration. This aberration increases between the first and third premature beats because of their prematurity.

Conclusion

    Atrial premature beats that are either blocked or conducted with aberrant conduction.

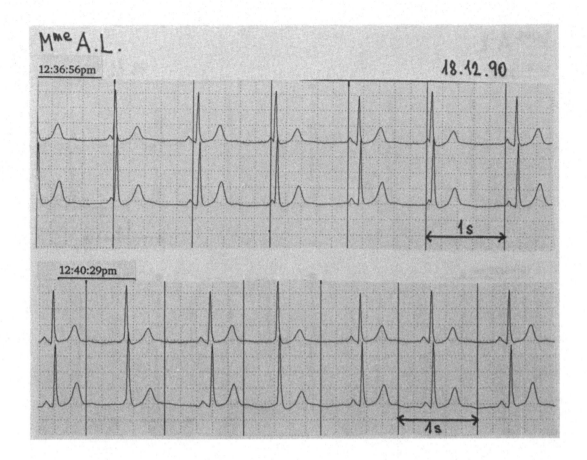

ECG no. 189: Mrs. A.L., 44 years

Status post cerebrovascular accident with aphasia
No medication
Holter ECG monitoring (two tracings at different times)

195

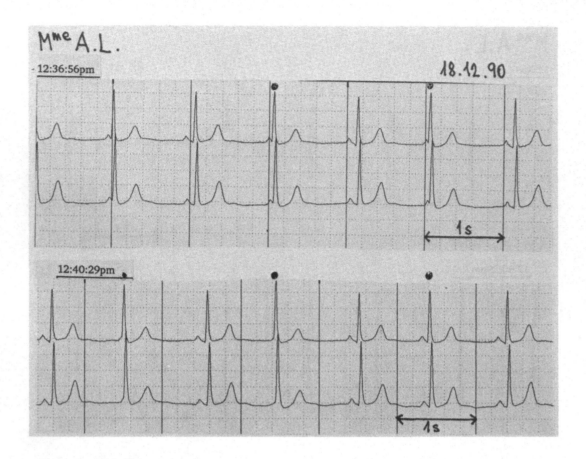

ECG no. 189: Mrs. A.L., 44 years

Holter ECG monitoring (two tracings at different times)

Upper tracing: At the atrial level, sinus rhythm is present. The QRS complexes are narrow but not regular and sometimes follow the previous P waves too closely. Each QRS complex with a conducted sinus P wave is followed by an AV junctional beat (•). The R–R interval between the junctional beats stays the same, suggesting junctional parasystole.

Lower tracing: The junctional activity is slightly faster and responsible for the ventricular complexes represented by a dot (•). The other complexes are conducted sinus beats.

Conclusion

Sinus rhythm and enhanced junctional activity, suggesting parasystole.

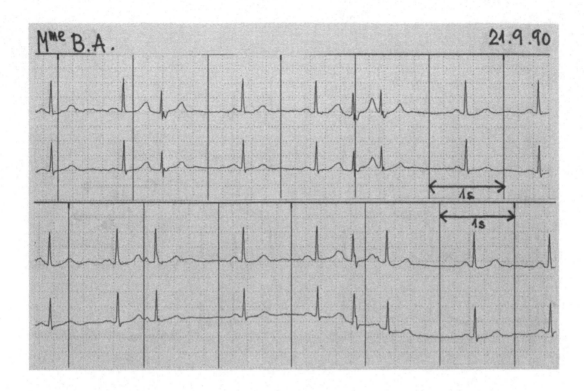

ECG no. 190: Mrs. B.A., 53 years

Palpitations
No treatment
Holter ECG monitoring (two noncontinuous tracings)

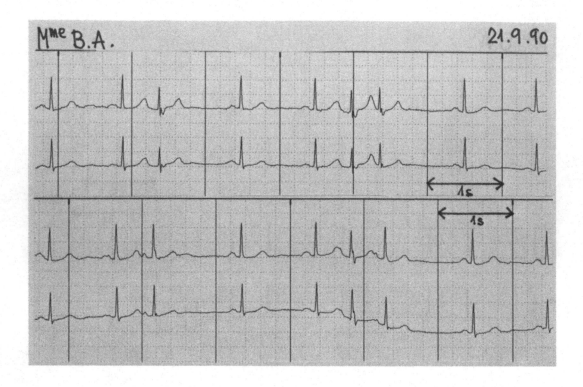

ECG no. 190: Mrs. B.A., 53 years

Holter ECG monitoring (two noncontinuous tracings)

Upper tracing: Sinus rhythm with occasionally wide QRS complexes. They are located after the second sinus complex, and twice following the fourth sinus complex. The T waves of the complexes preceding these beats are fuller and bigger, indicating atrial premature beats. They are conducted to the ventricle with intraventricular aberration.

Lower tracing: Again, atrial premature beats are visible but less premature; therefore, they show less intraventricular aberration.

Conclusion

Atrial extrasystoles with wide QRS complexes due to an intraventricular aberration.

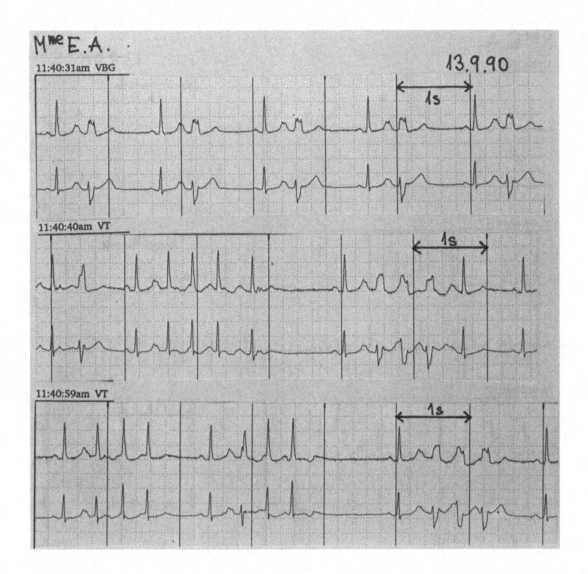

ECG no. 191: Mrs. E.A., 58 years

Many episodes of malaise with impression of loss of consciousness
No treatment
Three Holter ECG tracings

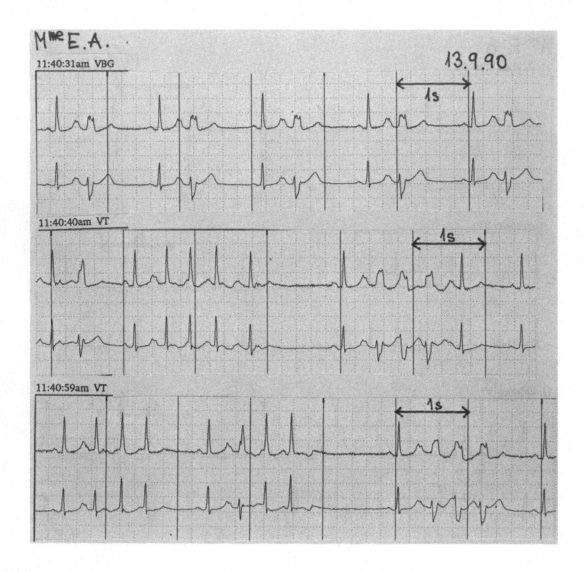

ECG no. 191: Mrs. E.A., 58 years

Three Holter ECG tracings

Top tracing: Wide QRS bigeminy. The T waves indicate the presence of atrial premature beats conducted with aberrant intraventricular conduction.

Middle tracing: Two irregular atrial tachycardias (of four QRS each). In the second tachycardia, the first three complexes are wider than the fourth one.

Bottom tracing: Three runs of irregular atrial tachycardia (of three complexes each) with different degrees of aberrant intraventricular conduction.

Conclusion

Sinus rhythm with frequent ectopic atrial activity showing different degrees of intraventricular conduction aberration.

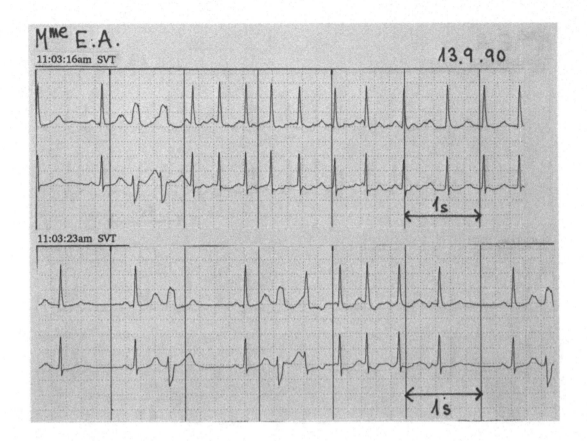

ECG no. 192: Mrs. E.A., 58 years

Many episodes of malaise with impression of loss of consciousness
No treatment
Two Holter ECG tracings

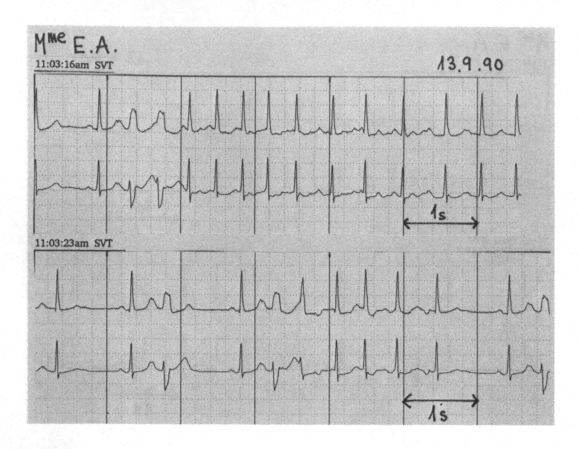

ECG no. 192: Mrs. E.A., 58 years

Two Holter ECG tracings

Upper tracing: Sinus rhythm is followed by rapid irregular ventricular activity because of AV conduction during atrial fibrillation. The first two QRS complexes are wide because of intraventricular aberration.

Lower tracing: Two conducted sinus beats are followed by an aberrantly conducted atrial premature beat. Thereafter, we see the onset of atrial fibrillation, the first two complexes with intraventricular aberration.

Conclusion

Atrial premature beats and runs of atrial fibrillation with intraventricular conduction aberration.

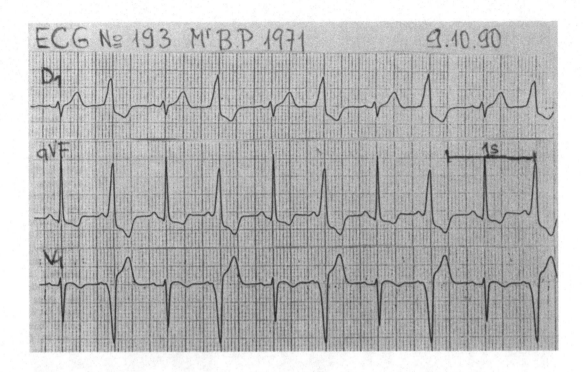

ECG no. 193: Mr. B.P., 19 years

Palpitations
No treatment
Leads I, aVF, and V_1

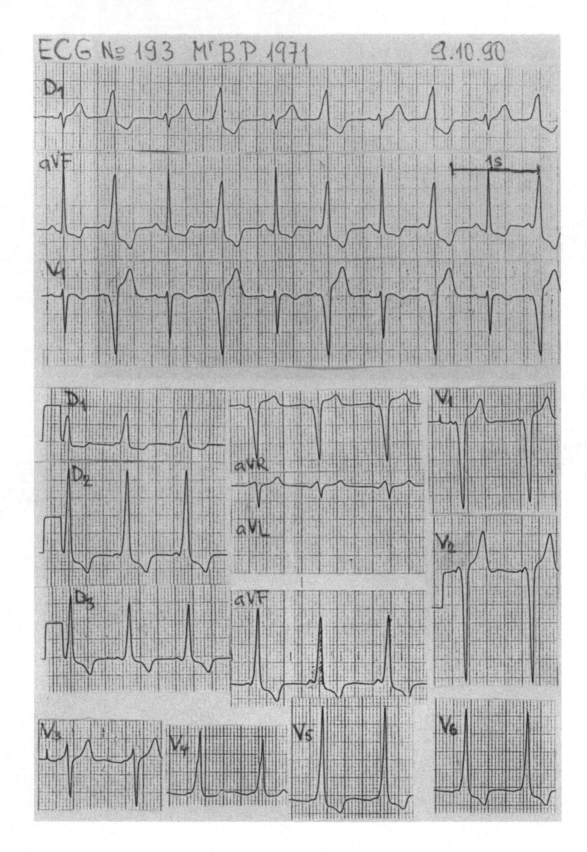

ECG no. 193: Mr. B.P., 19 years

Leads I, aVF, and V$_1$

Normal sinus rhythm. The ventricular complexes show alternating narrow and wide QRS. The narrow QRS is a conducted sinus beat. The wide QRS complex has a left bundle branch block configuration and is preceded by a sinus P wave with a short to the QRS. The differential diagnosis is late coupled ventricular beats arising in the right ventricle versus intermittent ventricular preexcitation. The latter diagnosis is suggested by the small delta wave seen in lead V$_1$. No definite diagnosis can be made with these three leads. The 12-lead ECG clearly shows that the correct diagnosis is ventricular preexcitation because of an anteroseptally located accessory AV pathway. In the 12-lead ECG, the sinus rate is somewhat slower than in the three-lead recording, allowing 1:1 conduction over the accessory pathway.

Conclusion

Intermittent (rate-related) Wolff–Parkinson–White (WPW) syndrome.

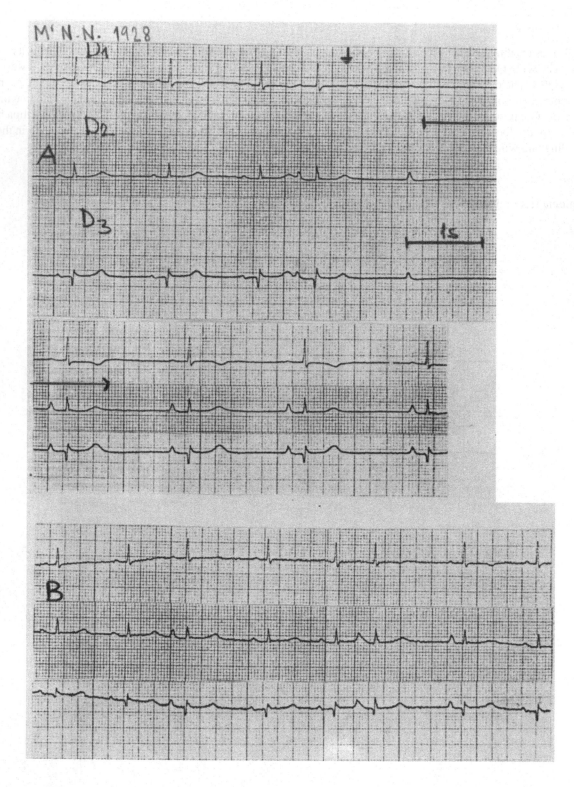

ECG no. 194: Mr. N.N., 62 years

Malaise
Syncope
No treatment

Tracing A: This is a continuous tracing; the *arrow* (↓) indicates the beginning of the right carotid massage.
Tracing B: The same leads (I, II, and III) were used, and this tracing was recorded after very mild exercise.

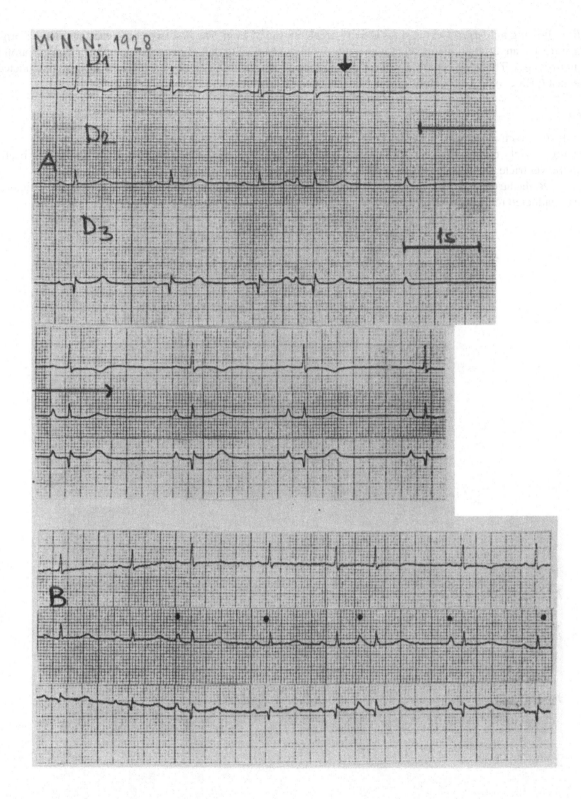

ECG no. 194: Mr. N.N., 62 years

Tracing A: The sinus bradycardia (~50 bpm) is followed after the third QRS by an atrial premature beat with a P wave morphology different from that of the three sinus P waves. Right carotid massage (↓) blocks the sinus activity, but the ectopic atrial activity persists, with a rate of 40 bpm. The first ectopic atrial beat is blocked, but the next four ectopic P waves conduct to the ventricles with a PR interval of 0.24 s. The ventricular complexes remain identical.

Tracing B: Following mild exercise, the sinus activity accelerates to 65 bpm. The first two complexes are of sinus origin, but then we again have an atrial premature beat with a morphology identical to that of the atrial complexes during carotid sinus massage in *tracing A*. The same ectopic P wave, now conducted to the ventricle, is present after the next two conducted sinus beats. The last QRS complex is of sinus origin.

Conclusion

We are dealing with atrial parasystole.

On *tracing A*, right carotid massage blocks sinus node activity. The atrial parasystole, apart from the first beat, is not blocked to the ventricle, but its rate is decreased by the massage.

On *tracing B*, the atrial parasystole (•) activates the atria when it occurs outside the refractory period of the sinus P wave and is then conducted to the ventricle.

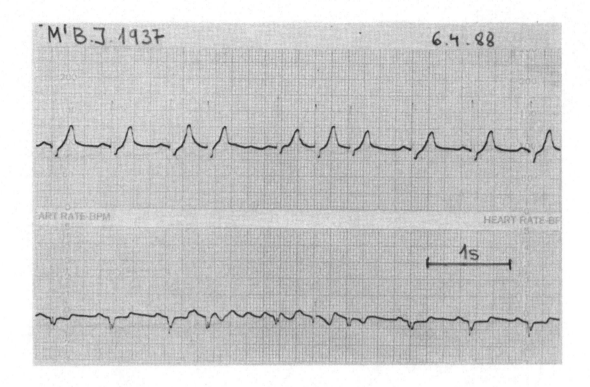

ECG no. 195: Mr. B.J., 51 years

Paroxysmal palpitations
ECG Holter recording

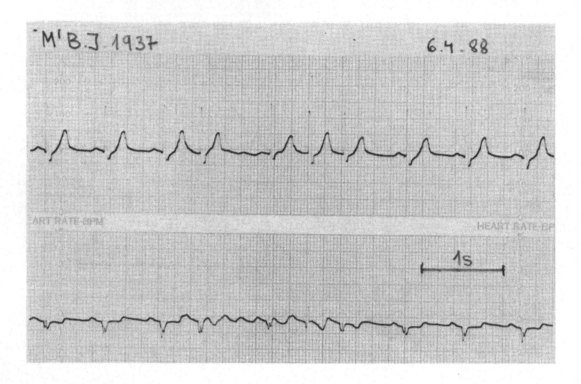

ECG no. 195: Mr. B.J., 51 years

ECG Holter recording

   The first three complexes are of sinus origin; they are followed by a fast atrial rhythm with the morphology of atrial flutter, with a rate of 300 bpm. The conduction to the ventricles is irregular. Normal sinus rhythm is present again in the last three complexes.

Conclusion

   Atrial flutter lasting no more than 2 s.

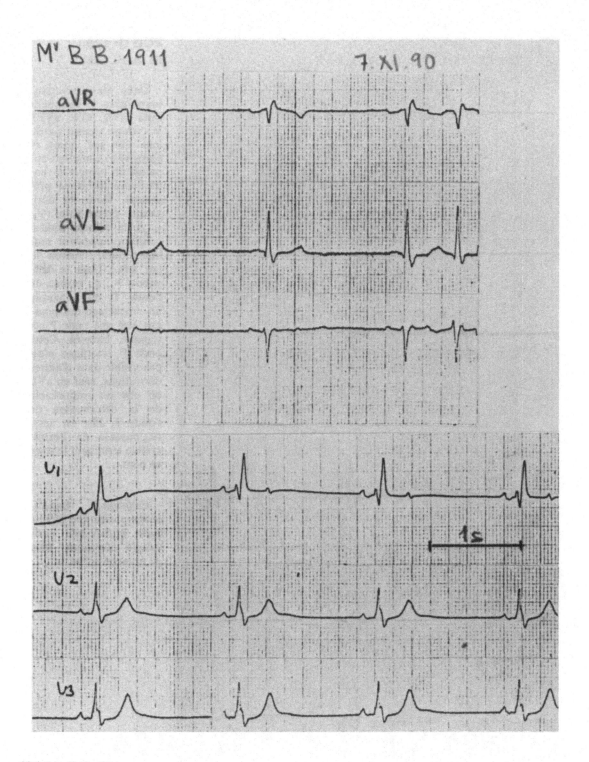

ECG no. 196: Mr. B.B., 79 years

Palpitations
Malaise
Heart insufficiency
Digoxin treatment, 0.125 mg, 5 days/week

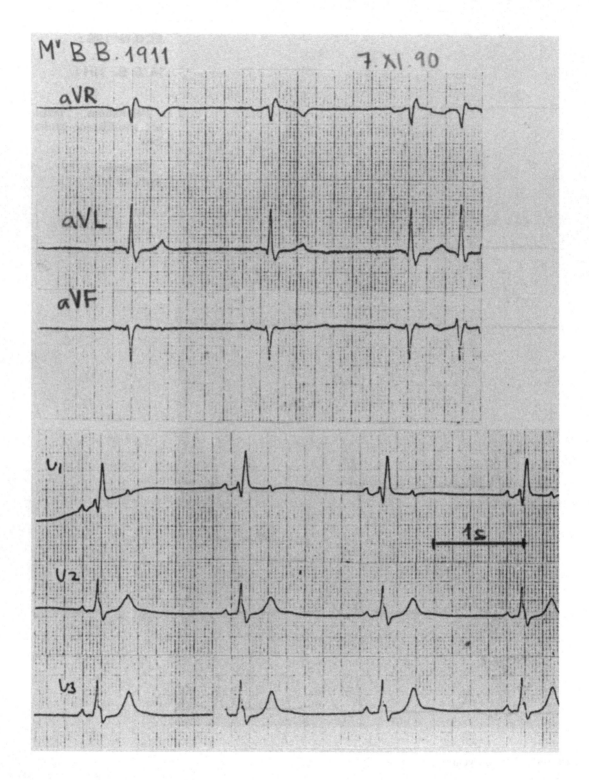

ECG no. 196: Mr. B.B. 79 years

In unipolar leads aVR, aVL, and aVF, a sinus bradycardia (40 bpm) is present. Nonconducted atrial premature beats are present in the T wave of the first two QRS complexes. There is also an ectopic P wave after the third complex, which is conducted to the ventricle with the same right bundle branch block configuration. The nonconducted coupled atrial premature beats are better seen in precordial leads V_1, V_2, and V_3.

Conclusion

Blocked atrial bigeminy with a single conducted premature beat at the end of the *upper tracing*; complete right bundle branch block.

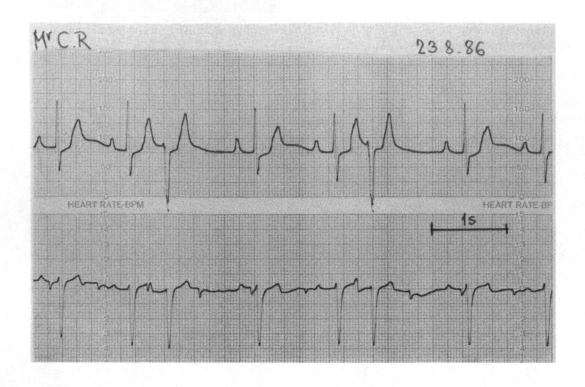

ECG no. 197: Mr. C.R., 52 years

Palpitations
Coronary artery disease
Holter ECG recording

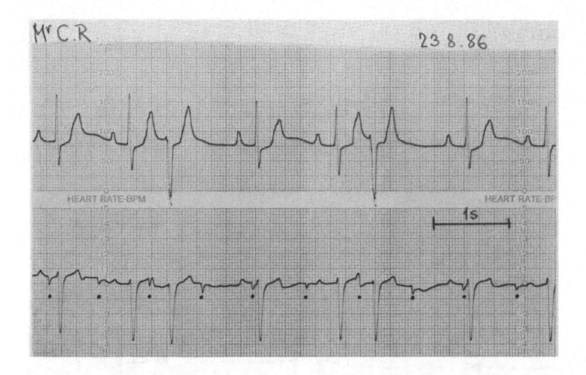

ECG no. 197: Mr. C.R., 52 years

Holter ECG recording

Normal sinus rhythm with atrial premature beats in the T wave after the second and fifth QRS. These premature beats are conducted to the ventricle with aberrant intraventricular conduction. In the inferior lead, the tracing presents regular notches because the magnetic tape (•) was insufficiently erased, resulting in artifacts from a previous recording.

Conclusion

Atrial trigeminy with intraventricular aberration. In the lower lead, there are artifacts due to insufficient erasing of the magnetic tape.

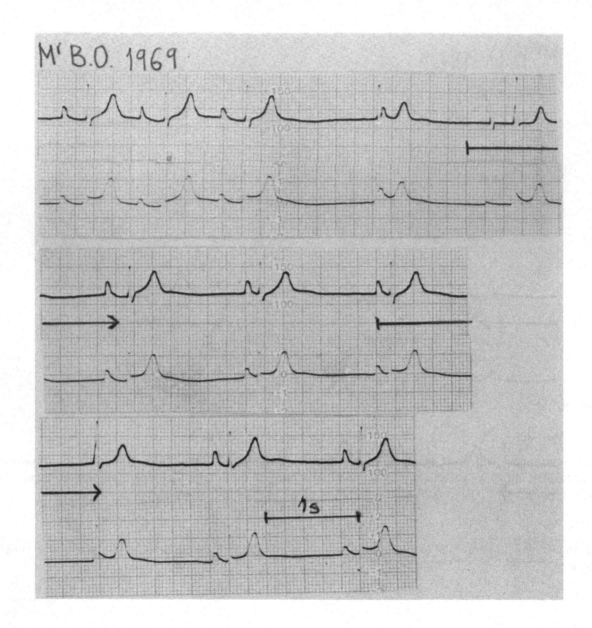

ECG no. 198: Mr. B.O., 21 years

Trisomy
Malaise
Holter ECG continuous recording

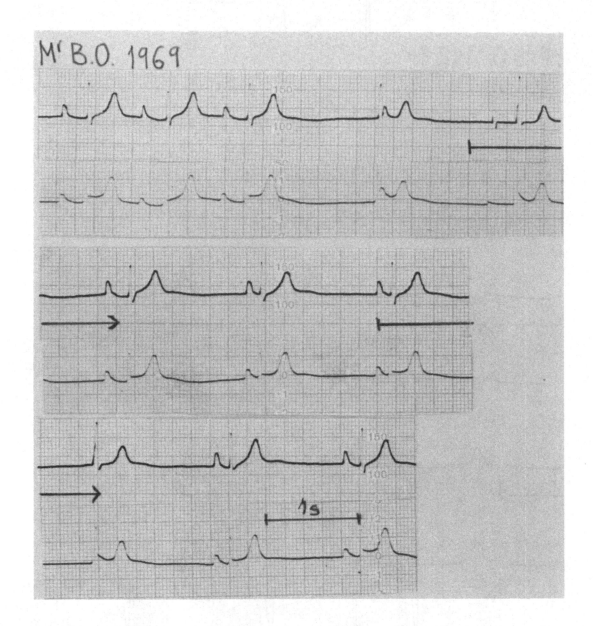

ECG no. 198: Mr. B.O., 21 years

Holter ECG continuous recording

Top strip: Sinus rhythm with prolonged PR is present in the first three beats, followed by two junctional escape beats.

Middle strip: Three beats of severe sinus bradycardia are present. They are followed in the *lower strip* by a junctional escape and two bradycardic sinus beats.

Conclusion

   Sick sinus syndrome with junctional escapes.

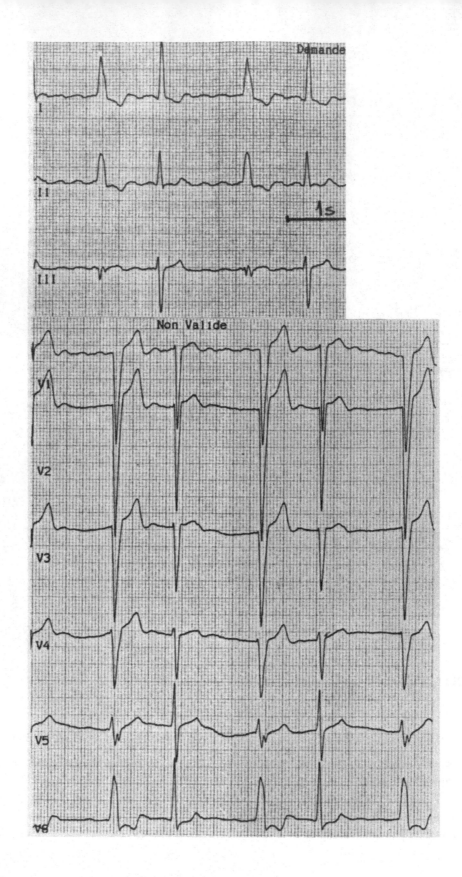

ECG no. 199: Mr. D.H., 61 years

Palpitations
Heart failure
Coronary artery disease
Digoxin treatment, 0.125 mg/day

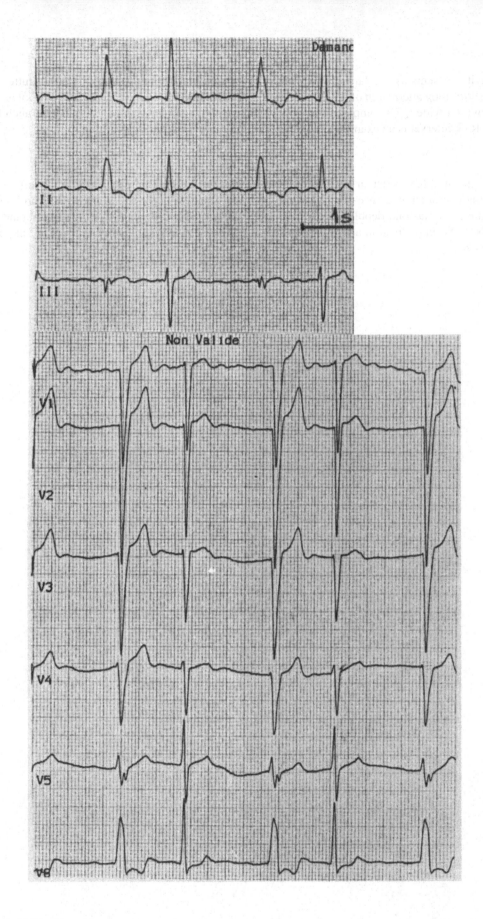

ECG no. 199: Mr. D.H., 61 years

The atrial activity presents as regular f waves with a rate of around 320 bpm, suggesting atrial flutter. The ventricular complexes show short–long alternation of the R–R interval. The short interval ends with a narrow QRS of around 100 ms and the long interval with a wide QRS complex of around 120 ms, with a configuration of left bundle branch block. The wide QRS after a long R–R interval is an example of phase 4 block in the left bundle branch.

Conclusion

Atrial flutter with variable ventricular conduction; after a long R–R interval, phase 4 block in the left bundle branch.

NB: Phase 4 bundle branch block is explained as follows. When phase 4 of the action potential is prolonged because of a long pause, spontaneous diastolic depolarization diminishes the potential difference with the membrane potential of the bundle branch fibers. When activation arrives, these fibers, being less polarized, cannot conduct the impulse, resulting in bundle branch block.

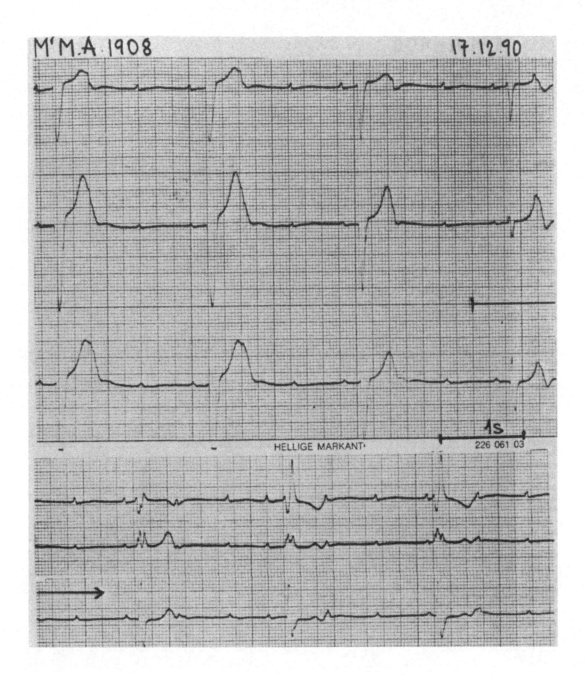

ECG no. 200: Mr. M.A., 82 years

Malaise
Loss of consciousness
No treatment
Leads V_1, V_2, and V_3
Continuous recording

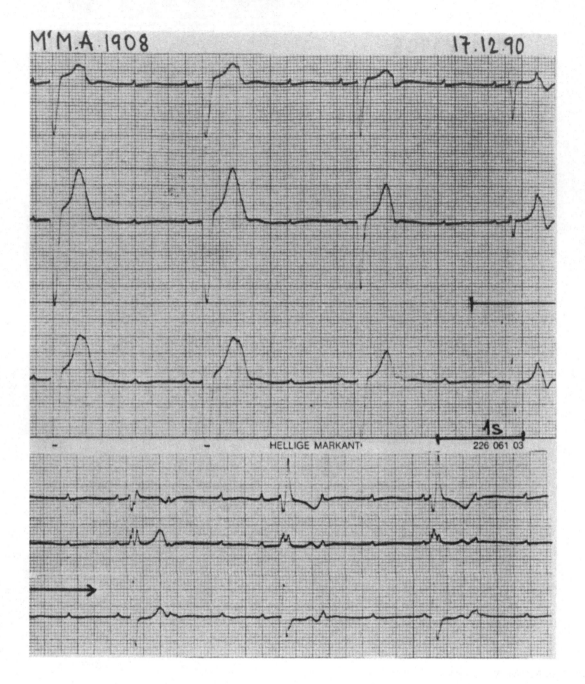

ECG no. 200: Mr. M.A., 82 years

Leads V_1, V_2, and V_3

Continuous recording

At the atrial level, sinus P waves are present with a rate of 100 bpm. No conduction is present between the atrium and ventricle. The ventricular complexes have different morphologies. The first two complexes are wide (0.14 s) and present a morphology of left bundle branch block. The third QRS has the same morphology but is slightly narrower at 0.12 s. The fourth QRS has a normal configuration and a duration of 0.10 s. The morphology of the fifth QRS complex changes into a

222

right bundle branch block pattern (0.12 s). The last two QRS complexes have a typical right bundle branch block configuration and a width of 0.14 s. The distance between the ventricular complexes shortens slightly, from 1,840 ms for the first two complexes to 1,760 ms for the last complexes. This increase in ventricular rate explains the change in QRS configuration. At the slower rate, the escape mechanism is in the right bundle branch, resulting in a left bundle branch block QRS configuration. The gradual change to a right bundle branch block with fusion QRS complexes in between (QRS 4 even having a normal QRS width!) is because a slightly faster escape mechanism in the left bundle branch takes over.

Conclusion

Complete AV block with competition at the ventricular level between two escape sites in the right and left bundle branches, respectively, with slight differences in the escape rate from these two sites.

Index

About the Authors

Dr. Richard Adamec received his medical doctor (MD) degree in 1957 from Charles University in Prague. In 1988, he became a privatdozent. From 1975 to 1979, he was senior registrar at the Cardiology Centre of the University Hospital of Geneva. From 1979 to 1998, he served as staff cardiologist at both the Geneva Medical University Policlinic and the Cardiology Centre of the University Hospital of Geneva. Between 1975 and 1998, he was responsible for interpreting all Holter ECG recordings performed at both those institutions.

Dr. Jan Adamec received his Swiss Medical Federal diploma in 1988 and his doctorate in medicine (MD) from Geneva University in 1994. Since 1996, he has served as an FMH Specialist in Cardiology and Internal Medicine. Since 1997, he has been a consultant cardiologist at the Cardiology Centre (University Hospital of Geneva); an associate cardiologist at the Cecil Clinic Hirslanden, Lausanne; and consultant cardiologist at the Clinic La Prairie, Montreux, Switzerland.

Dr. J.J. Hein Wellens, considered the founding father of clinical arrhythmology, studied medicine at the University of Leiden. From 1973 to 1977, he was professor of Cardiology at the University of Amsterdam. From 1977 to 2001, he served as professor of Cardiology and Chairman of the Department of Cardiology at the Academic Hospital of Maastricht University, creating a school of arrhythmology that educated more than 130 cardiologists from around the world during his tenure. Dr. Wellens also directed the Interuniversity Cardiological Institute of the Netherlands (ICIN) from 1993 to 2003 and was associate editor of Circulation from 1993 to 2004. He has authored or coauthored more than 600 peer-reviewed articles, 240 book chapters, and 20 cardiology books.